THE HISTORY
AND FUTURE OF
BIOETHICS

The History
and Future of
Bioethics

A Sociological View

John H. Evans

OXFORD
UNIVERSITY PRESS

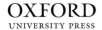

OXFORD
UNIVERSITY PRESS

Oxford University Press is a department of the University of Oxford.
It furthers the University's objective of excellence in research, scholarship,
and education by publishing worldwide.

Oxford   New York
Auckland   Cape Town   Dar es Salaam   Hong Kong   Karachi
Kuala Lumpur   Madrid   Melbourne   Mexico City   Nairobi
New Delhi   Shanghai   Taipei   Toronto

With offices in
Argentina   Austria   Brazil   Chile   Czech Republic   France   Greece
Guatemala   Hungary   Italy   Japan   Poland   Portugal   Singapore
South Korea   Switzerland   Thailand   Turkey   Ukraine   Vietnam

Oxford is a registered trade mark of Oxford University Press
in the UK and certain other countries.

Published in the United States of America by
Oxford University Press
198 Madison Avenue, New York, NY 10016

© Oxford University Press 2012

First issued as an Oxford University Press paperback, 2014.

Library of Congress Cataloging-in-Publication Data
Evans, John Hyde, 1965-
The history and future of bioethics : a sociological view / John H. Evans.
p. ; cm.
Includes bibliographical references and index.
ISBN 978-0-19-986085-2 (hardcover); 978-0-19-939705-1 (paperback)
1. Bioethics—History. I. Title.
[DNLM: 1. Bioethics—history. 2. Bioethics—trends. 3. History, 20th Century.
4. History, 21st Century. WB 60]
QH332.E93 2012
174.2—dc23
2011017268

9 8 7 6 5 4 3 2 1

Printed in the United States of America
on acid-free paper

CONTENTS

PREFACE

Social scientists teach their students the advantages and disadvantages of personal experience in social science research. On one hand, a native in a culture can investigate that culture in greater detail because they speak the language, both literally and metaphorically. They understand the basics, do not waste their time on obvious issues, and can really get to the real questions. An example of this model would be a devout Catholic conducting an ethnography of a Catholic church. On the other hand, an outsider to a culture can look at what would be mundane to the insider with fresh eyes— one could send an Orthodox Jew to conduct that ethnography of the Catholic church. They risk focusing on the obvious and well-known and ultimately uninteresting features of a culture. But, their fresh eyes make them question the ordinary events, which will be overlooked by the cultural insider.

What you have before you is a book written by a cultural outsider. Unlike the authors of most of the other texts available that reflect on the history, troubles, or solutions to the troubles of bioethics, I have never conducted an ethical consult, served on an institutional review board, had or taught a class in bioethics, served on a government ethics commission, been a member of a bioethics center, or even made a strictly ethical contribution to a public debate about science and medicine. Like the Orthodox Jew who wonders why those Catholics wave their hands over wine and bread every Sunday, it is my hope that I can look at what seems ordinary to insiders and question it. For example, while bioethicists take it for granted that they should be on federal bioethics commissions, I ask, by what authority do they claim legitimacy to do this? From this outside perspective I have created a fairly unorthodox history of bioethical debate and an unorthodox set of suggestions for resolving the current crisis in bioethical debate. Like ethnographies produced by religious outsiders, there will be parts of my analysis where insiders will feel that I have missed the mark due to a lack of intimate familiarity, but I hope there are enough fresh insights to make the reading worthwhile.

That said, I have been investigating bioethics as an outsider for a while now. Over the past 12 or more years I have had the privilege of being asked to speak at conferences or write papers on the topic of the structure of debates in bioethics. These talks and texts built upon my book that is broadly on this topic, *Playing God? Human Genetic Engineering and the Rationalization of Public Bioethical Debate* (2002).

I thank audiences at the Hastings Center; the American Society for Bioethics and Humanities Conference titled "Bioethics and Politics: The Future of Bioethics in a Divided Democracy"; the Center for American Progress; the Yale Interdisciplinary Bioethics Project, Yale University; the Social Trends Institute; the Society for Christian Ethics; the Center for Bio-medical Ethics and Department of Religion, University of Virginia; the Science and Religion Seminar Series of the Center for the Study of Science and Religion, Columbia University; the Center for Bioethics, University of Pennsylvania; Institution for Social and Policy Studies, Yale University; the Conference on the Twentieth Anniversary of the Belmont Report: the Past and Future Directions, University of Virginia; the Conference on Power, Interests, and Conflict in the Secularization of American Public Life, University of North Carolina, Chapel Hill; and on two separate occasions, the Economic and Social Research Council Genomics Forum at the University of Edinburgh.

As I wrote the various talks, I could feel that I had an overarching, broader narrative to tell than had been expressed in my 2002 book. I later decided to expand this broader narrative into the book you have before you. Some of these talks and texts had been printed in journals and edited volumes, and after sketching out the overall argument I wanted to make, I realized that some of the pieces of the overall argument had been well said in these publications. Not needing to reinvent the wheel, this book contains paragraphs taken from a few predecessor texts. I am grateful to the publishers for permission to reprint some paragraphs.[1] In addition to the audiences described above, and the reviewers and editors of the publications described immediately above, others deserve special thanks. The Department of Sociology at the University of California, San Diego has provided a great space for work like this. My longtime friend, the political theorist Mark Brown, deserves special thanks for a close reading of the manuscript at an early stage. His suggestions improved the manuscript markedly—although I do not doubt that I erred in ignoring some of his suggestions, and that we probably disagree about some issues. Confirming the power of an outsider view, another friend, Ben Hurlbut, provided an early in-depth critique by helping me understand the claims my own previous work had made. Elena Aronova, Laura J. Harkewicz, and Cathy Gere also provided incisive comments on an early draft of the entire manuscript. Reviewers from the press provided thorough comments on the entire manuscript, stopping me from making some fundamental errors. Finally, presentations of the argument of the entire book at the University of Pennsylvania Bioethics Center and the Center for Medical Ethics and Health Policy at Baylor College of Medicine were very helpful. At the University of Pennsylvania, thanks to Jonathan Moreno for sponsoring me, and Jonathan, Chuck Bosk, and David Grazian for helpful suggestions. At Baylor, thanks for Baruch Brody and Larry McCullough for sponsoring me. I have no doubt that many of those who graciously commented upon drafts of this book will remain in disagreement about at least some of my claims, and that any remaining errors are my own.

Notes

1. Four paragraphs in the introduction and three-quarters of Chapter 1 are taken from "After the Fall: Attempts to Establish an Explicitly Theological Voice in Debates over Science and Medicine after 1960," pp. 434–461 in *The Secular Revolution: Power, Interest, and Conflict in the Secularization of American Public Life*, edited by Christian Smith (Berkeley: University of California Press, 2003). Chapter 1 also includes approximately six paragraphs from "The Tension Between Progressive Bioethics and Religion," pp. 119–141 in *Progress in Bioethics: Science, Policy and Politics*, edited by Jonathan D. Moreno and Sam Berger (Cambridge, Mass.: MIT Press, 2010).

Chapter 2 contains approximately nine paragraphs from "After the Fall," approximately 25 paragraphs from "A Sociological Account of the Growth of Principlism" (*The Hastings Center Report* 30 [5]: 31–38, 2000), and six paragraphs from "Science, Bioethics and Religion," in *The Cambridge Companion to Science and Religion*, edited by Peter Harrison (Cambridge, UK: Cambridge University Press, 2010). Chapters 4 and 5 contain approximately six paragraphs from "Between Technocracy and Democratic Legitimation: A Proposed Compromise Position for Common Morality Public Bioethics" (*Journal of Medicine and Philosophy* 31 [3]: 213–234, 2006).

INTRODUCTION

Every day we hear of a new development in science, technology, and medicine, such as cloning, organ replacement, embryonic stem cell research, human genetic engineering, and reproductive genetic technology. This list is in many ways already dated, as science has produced more cutting-edge issues. To give but a few of many examples, it is now apparently possible to create embryos that are hybrids between cows and humans, and scientists are also trying to create, through what is now called *synthetic biology*, a "minimal chassis" of a life form, onto which could be attached building blocks that produce useful functions.

Few citizens would say that scientists should do whatever they want to do, and most people would say that we should have some sort of collective oversight over how these technologies evolve. But, how to do it? The most obvious answer, and the most institutionalized, is that there should be government rules about how scientific research is conducted and what research can be done. For example, scientists must ask the permission of people that they experiment upon, and there remain restrictions on what scientists can do with embryos (at least with government money.)

Professionally Mediated Debate
in the Public Sphere

The rules are created by government officials, and in principle, the government makes rules after listening to the voice of the citizens in the "public sphere," which I define, following Charles Taylor, as "a common space in which the members of society are deemed to meet through a variety of media: print, electronic, and also face-to-face encounters; to discuss matters of common interest; and thus to be able to form a common mind about these" (Taylor 1995: 185–186). In principle, the citizens debate each other, weed out the bad arguments, and come to some modicum of consensus that is transmitted to the state and acted upon. For example, there seems to be a consensus in the public sphere that reproductive cloning is bad, and our government officials are aware of this consensus, and have created policies to see that this is not allowed, at least with government money. There seems to be a social consensus that organ donation, but not selling, is acceptable. On other issues, such as abortion, the public mind does not seem to form one opinion.

Much of the debate in the public sphere is unmediated. We talk with the neighbors over the fencepost about the problem of rowdy neighborhood parties and what, if anything, the government should do about it. On other issues, social movements and interest groups organize and promote certain positions and collectively present these perspectives to our elected officials. For example, the American Association of Retired Persons (AARP) lobbies the government to promote the interests of its members in health-care policy.

There is an entire class of issues in the public sphere where some people have more authority to speak than others, and gatekeepers of discourse in the public sphere—like the editors of newspapers—give these people a bigger soapbox that allows them to shape the debate, and government officials listen more closely to some citizens than others. For example, on the question of whether we should allow nuclear power plants, a central question is safety, and physicists who know a lot about nuclear energy are allowed by these gatekeepers to disproportionately shape the citizen's views by appearing on TV or be quoted in the newspaper. Government officials will also seek out their advice. The reason is that ordinary people do not know as much about nuclear power as they do about rowdy neighborhood parties. When it comes to the government's deciding whether to encourage nuclear power, we accept that nuclear physicists will have a particularly influential role in shaping, not only the views in the public sphere, but the public policy as well.

These influential people are professionals, and political scientist Albert Dzur summarizes the role of professions in the public sphere when he writes that "because of their specialized knowledge and claims to exclusive control over specific social problems, professions wield considerable power both inside their work environments and outside in public life . . . professions possess the power to distract, encourage, limit, and inform public recognition of and deliberation over social problems."[1]

Like nuclear power, biomedical technologies are also something that ordinary people are largely unfamiliar with. How, after all, does cloning work? Would a Hitler clone be evil? What is the relevant distinction between healing disease and genetically enhancing a person?

As with nuclear power, we have professionals who are experts in bioethical issues who are given bigger soapboxes by gatekeepers (like reporters). These experts inhabit an institution in the public sphere that I will call "cultural bioethics." These experts are sometimes also sought out by the government for advice. I call this institution "public policy bioethics."[2] These professionals are primarily academics who hold appointments in institutions of higher education. A general question in this sort of debate would be: Should the government allow scientists to create hybrid animal-human embryos?[3] Professionals have made ethical claims about this practice—pro and con.

This professional role is summarized well by the former chair of a federal bioethics commission, Edmund Pellegrino, who writes that "[b]ioethicists must take seriously their obligations as professed experts in the definition, analysis, and study of bioethical issues. This means giving attention first to what the public and its representatives cannot do without their help. This is to set out the issues as objectively as possible, provide sound arguments for competing positions, and present them publicly in a restrained and balanced way. . . . The bioethicist's purpose should be to provide the basis for the kind of moral considerations upon which good policy rests" (Pellegrino 2006:578).

Why should the reader care about a bunch of academics sitting at their desks scratching their heads with pencils? After all, they generally cannot make laws or policies themselves. The reason we should care is that these head-scratchers actually have a strong influence on what actually happens in medicine and science. They engage in what political scientists would call "agenda-setting" in the public sphere, defining the legitimate boundaries of public debates, identifying which ethical issues are "important" and which are not. Their conclusions have influence on what actually happens in the real world through two mechanisms—by directly or indirectly communicating with government officials who have the power to set policy on biomedicine, and through directly or indirectly communicating with the citizens, who in turn influence government officials. This agenda-setting is a great power—some would say it is the greatest power of all (Lukes 1974).

The Crisis of the Bioethics Profession

It is good to have professionals in the public sphere, and it is useful if there is a profession that can be looked to to share its expertise so that public debates can be improved. For example, physicists improve debates about nuclear power, and sociologists improve the debate about family structure. As I will discuss in greater detail below, there is a profession called "bioethics" that is looked to to improve the debates over biomedical and scientific issues. However, the health of the bioethics profession is in question.

On the one hand, its influence seems to be growing with leaps and bounds. In the words of Carl Elliott, "Bioethics is spreading like kudzu, colonizing new areas even where it is unfamiliar, unexpected, and unwelcome. It is generating new centers, new journals, new courses, new commissions, new funding sources, and perhaps most visibly, a newly politicized presence in American public life. Americans can hardly open a newspaper or watch television without encountering a so-called bioethics expert" (Elliott 2005:379). Similarly, others have noted that

> over the course of four decades, bioethics has come to be recognized as an authoritative field. . . . Increasingly, bio-ethicists are sought after for their expertise—in clinical research and in government, legal, corporate, and community contexts—by universities, hospitals, businesses, policy makers, and the media. The rising demand for the contributions of those professionals have spurred the growth of graduate programs and centers—both free standing and university based—devoted to the study and practice of bioethics (Eckenwiler and Cohn 2007:xix).

On the other hand, the profession is said to be in crisis. As the authors cited above continue, "as the field has matured, there has been considerable controversy and critique concerning its work and the behaviors of those doing the work" (Eckenwiler and Cohn 2007:xix). Similarly, in an editorial in the *Lancet*, the author writes:

> Hardly wet behind the ears, bioethics seems destined for a short lifespan. Conspiring against it is exposure of the funding of some of its US centres by pharmaceutical companies; exclusion of alternative perspectives from the social sciences; retention of narrow analytical notions of ethics in

the face of popular expression and academic respect for the place of emotions; divisions within the discipline (including over its origins and meaning); and collusion with, and appropriation by, clinical medicine (Cooter 2004).

Another scholar goes as far as to ask "does bioethics exist?" The reason for the question is that "as bioethics has acquired academic standing, institutional authority and public visibility, just what constitutes 'bioethics' is becoming increasingly murky" (Turner 2009:778). Can we imagine someone asking "does the legal profession exist?" or "does the medical profession exist?"

A great case study in the crisis of the bioethics profession came during the political debate over health-care reform in the summer of 2009, where the writings of bioethics professionals were used by conservatives to erode support for the Democrats' health plan. For example, former vice-presidential candidate Sarah Palin said that the Democrats' plan would result in squads that would euthanize children like her youngest child, who has Down's syndrome. The basis for these claims was a few select passages from the work of Ezekiel Emanuel, a bioethicist who works at the National Institutes of Health, who also happened to be the brother of President Obama's chief of staff.[4] Later, Republican officials described a health planning book written by a bioethicist and distributed by the government to veterans as a "death book" that "encourages veterans to kill themselves or forgo care."[5] In both cases, prominent bioethicists rushed out to defend their clearly defamed colleagues; such as Arthur Caplan, who wrote that the claims were "an exercise in ludicrous, inflammatory rhetoric."[6] The board of directors of the primary professional association of bioethicists, the American Society for Bioethics and the Humanities, issued a "response to the recent attacks on bioethicists," complaining about the inaccurate portrayals of the work of these bioethicists and the disservice to the society that the bioethicists "seek to serve," and declaring that the claims "denigrate bioethics as a profession."[7]

On the one hand, these attacks should be considered simple political opportunism. However, the fact that these attacks seem to resonate with conservatives tells how weak the bioethics profession is. Conservatives just do not seem to accept the bioethics profession, and no statement about the claims of bioethicists seems too wild to believe to a good portion of the population. What is worse, usually when political operatives want to delegitimize the claim of a professional, they need to find another person with the same professional status to do their dirty work. For example, politicians cannot critique climatology themselves, so advocates of the climatological status quo have to find other climatologists to make these challenges. In the case of Republicans and health-care, they did not even need to find a self-identified bioethicist to make the claim that Emanuel's writing implied death squads; they could just do it themselves. Stronger professions could not be so easily challenged by outsiders within the area in which they claim expertise.

Professions and the Crisis in Bioethical Debate

There is a legitimacy crisis for the bioethics profession, and the crisis is best understood through looking at bioethical debate as the locus of competition between a number of professions vying for what I will call "jurisdiction" over the task of making ethical claims about medical and scientific technologies and practices. I will use this idea of a competing system of professions as a central analytical lens, so more detail is necessary.

In his canonical text on the professions, Andrew Abbott conceptualizes the central phenomena of interest in the study of professions as "jurisdiction," the link professionals make between themselves and a series of tasks, or their "work" (Abbott 1988). For example, physicians have established the jurisdictional link between themselves and the act of cutting into bodies with knives to heal diseases. A profession has jurisdiction if the audience for the jurisdictional evaluation thinks it should. In the case of physicians, the primary audience is public opinion—people are convinced that physicians should have jurisdiction over surgery, not some other profession (such as lawyers). Similarly, we do not look to a physicist to prepare our estate plan, but a lawyer. In the cases examined in this book, who the jurisdiction-giver *is* is of critical importance for determining which profession has jurisdiction over bioethical debate.

More important, a profession obtains jurisdiction by having a "system of abstract knowledge" that legitimates its claim over certain tasks. Medicine, for example, has the system of abstract knowledge called *medical science*, which contains much knowledge about the reaction of the body to being cut by knives, as well as the definitions of and methods for curing disease. It is the legitimacy of using the system of abstract knowledge for the task in the eyes of the jurisdiction-givers that confers jurisdiction over that task. Physicians have increasing jurisdiction over reducing the weight of an obese person because the public as jurisdiction-giver thinks its system of abstract knowledge—medical science—is better for this task than a competing system of abstract knowledge, like that proposed by dieticians.

Professions do not simply take over and "professionalize" a task, but rather are in constant competition with each other for jurisdiction over the same tasks. Medicine has been in competition with chiropractic care over the task of relieving back pain, and has faced recent challenges on other tasks, from acupuncture and aroma therapy. Of course, medicine has been one of the most successful professions, competing for and winning jurisdiction over all sorts of tasks formerly under the jurisdiction of other professions, such as alcoholism, mental illness, and obesity. It is so successful that there is a special term for its voracious additions of jurisdiction—*medicalization* (Conrad 2007).

The final part of Abbott's work to consider for our purposes is that all of these competing professions and the tasks they are competing over are considered to be in a large ecological system. Changes in the entire environment of the system, such as the rise of the bureaucratic state as the audience and jurisdiction-giver, can lead to a reshuffling of the entire system of professions, because the new jurisdiction-giver has different criteria for a legitimate system of abstract knowledge.

Finally, other ecological metaphors can be helpful. For example, professions can concentrate their energy on one task to protect themselves, or spread themselves thinly in the interest of jurisdictional expansion. They can also spread themselves too thinly through jurisdictional expansion and threaten their jurisdiction in their once-secure jurisdictional homeland.

Some professions have absolutely rock-solid jurisdictions that face no credible threat. Medicine's core jurisdiction over healing disease in human bodies really faces no challengers, and it is so institutionalized that if a person not certified by the profession tries to engage in the task they will be thrown in jail by the government.

The task space of making ethical claims about scientific and medical technologies and practices has been a much less institutionalized area, with many professions fighting for jurisdiction over the past few decades. No profession has approached the level of institutionalized jurisdiction that medicine has over healing disease, but the nascent bioethics profession has had the most success. As I will describe in the next few chapters, in the 1960s, there was a struggle between, on one side, the related and cooperating professions of science and medicine, which I will often abbreviate as "science/medicine." (For my purposes they can be considered the same profession in that they have the same interests and, more important, use the same system of abstract knowledge when it comes to ethics.) On the other side was the profession of theology. More minor competitors in the early days were the professions of law, philosophy, and social science. In the 1960s, theology was trying to use its existing system of abstract knowledge to defend its jurisdiction over ethics from science/medicine. In the 1970s a new profession arose that I will call the "bioethics profession," which had a system of abstract knowledge that was designed to please the jurisdiction-givers. The profession gained jurisdictions.

A Bioethics Profession?

Many readers will balk at this point, claiming that there is no "profession" of bioethics, only bioethical debates comprising people from established professions. This claim is a holdover from the original vision of some of the earliest participants in bioethical debates, who *were* arguing for a pan-professional assault on the science/medicine profession's secure jurisdictions and jurisdictional expansion plans. However, there is now clearly a distinct profession called "bioethics."

First, there is a population of professionals who call themselves "bioethicists." Scholars who are continually quoted in the *New York Times* are referred to as "bioethicists" and not "philosophers," "lawyers," or some other professional identity. Academic centers devoted to the tasks that I argue the profession now has jurisdiction over call themselves "bioethics" centers, and not the "Center for Applied Philosophy" or the "Center for Biomedical Law." There is a professional association with the word *bioethics* in the title that releases statements about defending "bioethics as a profession."[8]

Of course, the profession of bioethics is not as institutionalized as others at this point in its short history (Baker 2009). Unlike medicine, it generally lacks an exact academic degree like the M.D., although M.A.s and Ph.D.s in bioethics are increasingly available. Because it is so new, all of the profession's founders and the majority of current practitioners were trained in other professions, like philosophy, law, or theology, so the distinct professional identity is often blurred. Moreover, many people doing the work of bioethics are doing so part-time, with their primary jobs being something like medicine, nursing or social work (Fox, Myers and Pearlman 2007:17).

While there is a professional association, debates continue about credentialing, a code of ethics, and other features of a more institutionalized profession (Scofield 2008; Baker 2009). It could also be argued that while there are people who call themselves "bioethicists," they are so eclectic that there is no way to say they are unified by one system of abstract knowledge (Turner 2009). However, I will argue that there *is* a unified system of abstract knowledge that defines the profession, and to the extent that there is not, there should be.

Remember that, in the sociological approach to the professions, professions are not defined by their associations or academic degrees, but by their systems of abstract knowledge. I will further flesh out the details of the bioethics system of abstract knowledge in subsequent pages. For now I will define *bioethicists* as professionals who use methods in a system of abstract knowledge wherein ethical recommendations are *not* based on their own personal values or the values of a particular group in society, but based on the values of either the individuals involved with an ethical decision or the values of the entire public. A professional is not a bioethicist if they make recommendations based upon their own values or the values of a subgroup of the public.[9] In political theorist Mark Brown's division of bioethicists into liberals, communitarians, and republicans, I am therefore defining all bioethicists as "liberals." (I would describe those in Brown's other categories as members of other professions competing with the bioethics profession.) And, as liberals, their central concept is that they do not want to impose their values on others: "Liberal bioethics thus models itself on a rationalist and decisionist view of expertise, according to which experts provide value-neutral knowledge that allows non-experts to effectively pursue their subjective preferences" writes Brown (Brown 2009:45).[10] (Please note that this political-theory form of liberalism does not correspond with the common use of "liberal" in politics. Right-wing Republicans can be liberals in the philosophical sense.) Other professions competing with bioethics, such as theology and science (see Chapter 2), either tended to or appeared to promote the values of a subgroup of the public.

My definition of the system of abstract knowledge of the bioethics profession is consistent with the understanding of most participants in these debates. The bioethicists' system of abstract knowledge is evident in bioethicists' work in hospitals, where they argue that they are primarily helping families and doctors clarify their own values so that families and doctors can make a decision that is right for them.[11] This system of abstract knowledge is evident in bioethicists' work in protecting the human subjects of research when they apply ethical principles that are purportedly taken from the "common morality," not from their own morality or the morality of a subgroup of the population. It is evident in government ethics commissions that try to foster consensus among diverse commissioners, because they argue that this means the ethical recommendations will represent the public's values.

The Revealing Debate about Bioethical Expertise

The bioethical literature on moral expertise reveals that my definition of the bioethics profession is consistent with the profession's self-understanding. (The early debates I describe below took place before the use of the term *bioethics* had solidified, so those I am calling bioethicists are often called "philosophers" in this debate.) The origin of this debate is the suspicion that there is no need for the profession at all because there is no such thing as ethical or moral expertise. Many people think that bioethical debate is like the debate about loud neighbors—everyone can have a legitimate opinion about what to do about the neighbors, and everyone can have a legitimate opinion about the morality of cloning. At one extreme is Shalit, who writes that, "if you take democracy seriously, then the basic rule is that every philosopher is simply a citizen, and every citizen a philosopher, capable of making decisions that reflect his or her conscientiously held beliefs."[12] In short, the argument is that bioethicists have no more expertise than any citizen and should not be allowed a platform with which to speak that is not allowed to the ordinary citizen.

This strong argument taken against bioethicists as moral experts is that, for "moral expertise" to exist, there must be moral facts, and there must be objective answers about right and wrong. There must be "an agreed-upon set of facts and criteria" (Yoder 1998:13)— a true right and wrong that would not vary by culture, ethnic group, religion, and so on, with one true answer that a bioethicist could in principle discern.

However, Yoder points out that this is a straw man, in that "those who think there is ethical expertise . . . deny that they ever claimed to have *that type* of expertise" (Yoder 1998:13). Yoder goes on to cite bioethicist John Fletcher that "the goal of clinical ethics is to help clinicians and other professionals develop the ability to 'identify, understand, and help resolve ethical problems that arise in clinical practice'" (Yoder 1998:13). Similarly, Yoder, quoting Crosthwaite, argues that:

> expert ethical opinions flow from the proper employment of three sorts of philosophical expertise—skills, knowledge, and values. The skills are the ability to clarify and analyze concepts and problems and the ability to construct and assess arguments. The knowledge is of philosophical problems, questions, and theories; of assumptions and consequences of different positions; and of types of arguments and fallacies. The values include a commitment to understanding issues and views, a commitment to reasoned support and evolution of claims, a willingness to question assumptions and received wisdom, and an interest in finding solutions to philosophical questions (Yoder 1998:13).

Note that the values in the above statement are not those of the bioethicist.

Peter Singer, responding to a writer who claims there is no relevant ethical expertise, writes that philosophers have no expertise in "the possession of special moral wisdom or privileged insights into moral truth, but in understanding the nature of moral theories and the possible methods of moral argument" (Singer 1982:9). Singer thinks that philosophers have a number of advantages. First, they have training in "logical arguments and detecting fallacies." Second, they have training in metaethics—"what it is to make a moral judgement." Third, they know theories like utilitarianism that are "often helpful in discussing practical ethical issues." Fourth, they can think about ethics full-time, while others have other jobs to do (Singer 1982:9–10).

Tom Beauchamp sees four contributions that philosophers can make. The first is "conceptual analysis," to forge agreement on terms like "research," and "human subject." A second is "exposing the inadequacies and unexpected consequences of an argument." Beauchamp uses the example of how some abortion arguments could logically be applied to infants. A third is engaging in collaboration with other professions to set policy, and a fourth is participation in institutional and policy decision making. He does not mention what specific contribution philosophers could make to these final two situations.[13]

Similarly, and more recently, R. Alta Charo sees bioethics as helping others clarify *their* values, writing that the field of bioethics "gained some of its credibility because it was thought to offer something distinctive: knowledge of ethical and political theory, as well as relevant law, and a commitment to analytical reasoning that helps others to articulate their assumptions and fundamental values and challenges others to develop positions that logically flow from those assumptions and values" (Charo 2007:98).

In a summary statement, Lillehammer writes that it is a misconception to think that bioethicists' claim to expertise is that they can come up with a one true answer. Rather, their expertise is a clarifying expertise:

> The role of bioethicists is vindicated by their possession of a critical and systematic mastery of ethical concepts and positions, of the presuppositions of such positions, and the relations and distinctions between them. It is in the application of this knowledge that philosophical expertise comes into its own right by encouraging a more informed level of debate in bioethics" (Lillehammer 2004:133).

There are very detailed debates about these various clarifying and qualifying skills of bioethicists, and the question is whether or not ordinary people have these same skills. That detailed question is unimportant to me, and I assume that bioethicists are better at these tasks than ordinary people. Critically, in all of the reading I have done on the claims of moral expertise by bioethicists, I have yet to encounter the claim that bioethicists are those who use their own values or the values of a subset of the citizens. Rather, they use the values of others. This is the core of their system of abstract knowledge, and they use multiple methods to discern, clarify, and use the values of others, depending on the context.

Rogue Bioethicists

An objection to my definition of the bioethics profession could be that Professor X, the most identifiable and famous person who calls herself a bioethicist, explicitly advocates values that she does not think of as held by the general public, but simply are "correct." In very recent years there has also emerged a group of professionals who are associated with a particular religious tradition who call themselves "Christian bioethicists" (Anspach 2010), who would not fit my definition because they are championing the values of a subgroup.

Again, the bioethics profession is not as institutionalized as medicine, where a physician who only uses "healing touch" would be thrown out of the profession. However, there *is* a dominant system of abstract knowledge and, importantly, to resolve the crisis there should be greater agreement among people who call themselves bioethicists on the system of abstract knowledge. To end the crisis in the jurisdictions of the bioethics profession, I will argue that Professor X and the Christian bioethicists should not call themselves bioethicists, but instead philosophers, theologians, or some other title. Clarifying this identity problem is the sort of "day of reckoning" that the bioethics profession has never faced, but it is what all professions must eventually do.

The reasons why professional titles like "bioethicist" must have some fixed meaning is pretty intuitive. If professions gain jurisdiction over task by their general reputation for their ability to work on tasks, determining which tasks a profession is known for is critical. If lawyers drew up wills, held court trials, negotiated divorces, constructed business leases, *and* designed valves in nuclear power plants, the public would ask, "why do I want someone with engineering knowledge of water flow, pressure per square inch, and the properties of metals to represent me in my divorce case?" Analogously, if "bioethicists" both help you clarify your own values *and* tell you what your own values should be, this will result in a lack of legitimacy for all bioethicists. Professions can soldier on for a long time with ambiguity, but eventually the tensions of not demarcating their own boundaries will come back to haunt them when their jurisdictions are attacked—which is what is happening to the bioethics profession now.

Finally, bioethicists also often object to the empirical claims of social scientists about the dominant system of abstract knowledge in the bioethics profession. However, this objection is voiced by the bioethical theoreticians, who do not recognize that their perspective is different from that of the professional masses. Every profession has its theoreticians, and their role is to argue about what the proper system of abstract knowledge of the profession should be. At this elite level, there *is* a debate between people who want the profession to adopt different systems of abstract knowledge based on pragmatism (McGee 1999), principlism (Beauchamp and Childress 2009), feminist bioethics (Tong 1997), casuistry (Jonsen and Toulmin 1988), and other theories. To give but one example, an article debating whether pragmatism should be the new system of abstract knowledge of the bioethics profession begins by claiming that the profession was "[d]ominated in the 1980s by so-called 'principlism' and utilitarian/deontological ethics," but "bioethics has turned to other perspectives" such as "narrative ethics, casuistry, and the ethics of care." "Like these other 'new' approaches, much has been made of late concerning the insurgence of pragmatism into both the clinical and theoretical aspects of the bioethics discipline" the author concludes (Hester 2003:545–546).

However, in the next paragraph the author acknowledges that, for pragmatism, one of these new systems of knowledge that is supposedly on par with principlism in the field, "there have been no standard textbooks in medical ethics that have included articles written from explicitly pragmatic perspectives" (Hester 2003:546). This suggests that, while all professions have theoreticians who argue over the proper system of abstract knowledge, the ordinary writers and practitioners of the bioethics profession are not followers of any of these challengers, but follow the methods and system of abstract knowledge I will describe in more detail below.

The Multiple Jurisdictional Claims of the Bioethics Profession

The existence of a distinct bioethics profession becomes even clearer through closely examining the task spaces that the profession competes for. The profession of bioethics seeks or defends jurisdiction over four related tasks.

The Health-Care Ethics Consultation Jurisdiction

The first task is health-care ethics consultation (American Society for Bioethics and Humanities 2011; Fox et al. 2006). As defined by the professional association of bioethicists, health-care ethics consultation is "a set of services provided by an individual or a group in response to questions from patients, families, surrogates, health-care professionals, or other involved parties who seek to resolve uncertainty or conflict regarding value-laden concerns that emerge in health-care" (American Society for Bioethics and Humanities 2011:4). This task is done by a committee, a team, or an individual. A typical question here would be whether life support should be ended for a patient when doctors and family members disagree.

The task of health-care ethics consultation itself is quite institutionalized. One study found that by the year 2000, 92% of hospitals with 100–199 beds had health-care ethics consultation, as did 100% of hospitals with more than 400 beds (Fox, Myers and Pearlman 2007:15). Moreover, the government regulator that accredits hospitals requires that hospitals have a process to handle ethical issues that arise, and a process is "legally mandated under specific circumstances in several states" (Fox et al. 2006:13). Another entity that establishes certification requirements for medical schools requires all medical schools to teach bioethics to their students.[14] The authors of one study conclude that health-care ethics consultation "has become a routine part of U.S. healthcare" (Fox, Myers and Pearlman 2007:19).

The vast majority of professionals who engage in this task are only part-time bioethicists (i.e., part-time users of the system of abstract knowledge). The rest of the time they are hospital employees engaged in other tasks. One study found that 34% were also physicians, 31% nurses, 11% social workers, 10% chaplains, 9% administrators, and fewer than 4% "other" professionals (which includes full-time self-identified "bioethicists.") (Fox, Myers and Pearlman 2007:17).

The system of abstract knowledge these part-time bioethicists are using is that of the bioethics profession. According to the report on core competencies for health-care ethics consultation published by the bioethics association, bioethicists are not to impose their own values, but rather to facilitate an ethical decision between the interested parties, constrained by what are called "established ethical standards" (American Society for Bioethics and Humanities 2011:45). While the phrase "established ethical standards" would not preclude using the ethics of some subset of the population, the practice is to use values portrayed as representing universal public morality, not the morality of some particular group.

I am aware of no challengers for jurisdiction over this task, and I consider this to be part of the secure jurisdictional homeland of the bioethics profession. To the extent that there is talk of crisis in this particular jurisdiction, it is from fear of shoddy work, not fear of a competing profession. Some of the challenges include the fact that the many tiny hospitals in the United States cannot afford to pay for health-care ethics consultation, that very few participants have formal training, and that ethics consults may be rare enough in small institutions that people cannot maintain their expertise (Fox, Myers and Pearlman 2007).

Research Bioethics Jurisdiction

The second jurisdiction of the bioethics profession is research bioethics, where the task is to propose ethical constraints on the behavior of individual scientists and physicians in scientific and medical research on humans. This task is even more institutionalized than health-care ethics consultation in that every entity that receives government research money must have an institutional review board to review the ethics of research conducted with federal funds. Nearly every institutional review board now reviews all research, whether federally funded or not. Like health-care ethics consultation, most of the bioethicists conducting this task are part-time and have other professional identities besides "bioethicist." For example, in a university, regular faculty members can be members of the institutional review board, as this is not a task that would require forty hours a week of work. Like health-care ethics consultation, the bioethicists' system of abstract knowledge is institutionalized, giving the profession nearly perfect jurisdiction. In fact, the jurisdiction over research bioethics is even more secure than over health-care ethics consultation, because the federal government enforces the use of the bioethicists' system of abstract knowledge through public regulation. In this jurisdiction, the "other people's values" that are being used are the general public's values, as the federal government requires the use of a particular method that claims to be using the public's universally held values.

As with health-care ethics consultation, I know of no challengers for jurisdiction over this task, and this is the other part of the safe jurisdictional homeland of the bioethics profession. While few question that bioethicists should have jurisdiction over the ethics of medical research on humans, attempts by bioethicists to expand this jurisdiction to include the task of evaluating the ethics of social science and humanities research have faced continued resistance (Bosk and DeVries 2004; Feeley 2007; Bosk 2010:S141). For example, some social scientists are debating whether to try to mount a constitutional challenge to institutional review board oversight of non-federally funded social science and humanities projects on the grounds that oversight is an infringement on free speech (Dingwall 2007; Katz 2007). But, again, the core of this jurisdiction is not under threat, and at worst the attempt to solidify an expanded jurisdiction over social science and humanities research may be thwarted.

Public Policy Bioethics Jurisdiction

The third task space is public policy bioethics. The task being competed over here is to propose ethical courses of action for scientists and physicians that can be incorporated into general policies that will be applied to all citizens. For example, the chair of one government ethics commission said the commission was created because "senior NIH administrators felt they needed guidelines to instruct members of Institutional Review Boards. . . charged with approving human subject and fetal tissue research" (Green 2001:3–4). This is the location of the crisis for the bioethics profession and is the primary but not exclusive focus of this book.

There are two sets of institutions that can enact ethical policy that would affect all citizens. The first is professional associations, such as the American Medical Association or the American Society for Reproductive Medicine. To the extent that a professional association's ethics policy is forced upon its members, and the members treat all the citizens, proposing ethical courses of action is in this jurisdiction. While I include these in my definition for inclusiveness, this task is a relatively minor part of this jurisdiction. A much larger proportion of bioethical activity is focused on the second type of institution—proposing ethical courses of action that can be incorporated into *government* policies, which are obviously applied to all citizens. In this book I will focus on the government as the primary "consumer" of suggested ethical policy.

This task of proposing ethics is carried out in many ways. Most influential is the government ethics commission, typically established by the executive branch to provide ethical advice (although states and the legislative branch have also established this mechanism).[15] For example, the recent President's Council on Bioethics had as its "principal aim" in one study "to describe and critically assess the various oversight and regulatory measures that now govern the biotechnologies and practices at the intersection of assisted reproduction, human genetics, and human embryo research" (Kass 2005:241). Similarly, James Lindemann Nelson writes that the outcomes of commissions "reasonably can be seen as assuming special normative authority, as well as an inside track to influencing the state's coercive powers" (Nelson 2005:254–255).

Testifying before Congress would also obviously fit in this task space, as would simply being asked for ethical advice by a government official who has the power to influence or set policy. For example, Leon Kass and Daniel Callahan were brought to the Oval Office and asked by President George W. Bush what was the most ethical course to pursue in embryonic stem cell research policy (Gamerman 2001).

Many professionals, including bioethicists, are working in this task space despite not being among the few who can serve on a commission or garner an audience with the president, by writing texts such as journal articles in order to influence a debate that ideally and eventually will be presented to government officials. The key to demarcating this task from the other task spaces is that the texts have to at least implicitly recommend policy that flows from the ethics, not simply state what is right or wrong. Of course, many academic texts blur this distinction, but we should keep the distinction in principle. So, most professionals in this task space are writing texts claiming, for example, that "the National Institutes of Health should fund experiments in germline human genetic engineering because of the following ethical reasons," or that "National Institutes of Health should not fund experiments" for some other ethical reason.

As with the other task spaces, the jurisdiction of the bioethics profession is obscured by the fact that many of the most visible bioethicists in this task space are part-time. For example, government ethics commissions have had a minority of members who would call themselves "bioethicists," and many have the identity of "scientist," "doctor," or "patient advocate." However, since the system of abstract knowledge of the bioethics profession is used to guide the conclusions of these commissions, the bioethics profession has jurisdiction here, too, regardless of the titles or self-identities of those using the system.

Jurisdiction is given by the audience for the task, and for this type of ethics, the audience is typically the unelected administrative agency employees who have to make policies (like whether government money can be used to create embryos for research). Elected officials have been somewhat less voracious consumers of this product. However, unlike health-care ethics consultation and research bioethics, the jurisdiction of the bioethics profession over this task, once fairly advanced, does appear to be in crisis in recent years, due to a change in the views of the jurisdiction-giver. I will elaborate on this below.

Cultural Bioethics Jurisdiction

The fourth task space I will call "cultural bioethics,"[16] which consists of trying to convince the ordinary citizens of the proper ethical course of action concerning a medical or scientific technology or practice. An example of this task would include being interviewed for a newspaper article and saying that reproductive cloning is wrong because it destroys the individuality of the clone. Another would be writing an article that concludes it is acceptable for scientists to destroy embryos to make stem cell lines because it is a moral imperative to heal disease. Communicating with the media, teaching, writing tracts intended for the public, and communicating through social-movement organizations are all tasks that professionals in this task space engage in. Most purely academic ethical writing that does not address policy would also fit into this category. This space is what social theorists consider to be the core of the public sphere, where the people debate among themselves—often mediated through the media and social movements—and the results of that debate are forwarded to the government for enactment through public opinion. Classically, enactment came through elections of our representatives, with the public, in theory, electing those who represented their views. Citizens' communication with elected officials, public-opinion polling, and other techniques also forward the conclusions of public debate to elected officials.

Obviously this cultural bioethics task space is difficult to demarcate in practice from public policy bioethics, in that many ethical claims implicitly or explicitly continue by saying that the government should create policy to support or oppose the use of some technology or practice. Moreover, government ethics commissions—a tool in the public policy task space—have often tried to act in both the public policy and cultural task spaces at once, speaking both to government officials and to the public. Yet, it is critical that we at least in principle try to detangle these two, because the lack of recognition of this boundary is one of the sources of the crisis for the bioethics profession. In a liberal democratic society, these two jurisdictions have different jurisdiction-givers, and, critically, they will not and should not accept the same system of abstract knowledge.

As I will describe in the next chapter, cultural bioethics was the first task space being fought over by myriad professions before the involvement of the government and before the advent of the bioethics profession. The bioethics profession has never gained jurisdiction over the cultural bioethics task, although it is one of the strongest contenders.[17] The jurisdiction-givers in this final jurisdiction are the gatekeepers of public discourse, like media reporters who decide which profession to give a soapbox to. We would recognize a 100% jurisdiction for the bioethics profession if every name in the Rolodex of science reporters under the heading "ethics of science/medicine" was someone who used the bioethics system of abstract knowledge. However, to the extent the gatekeepers need to be responsive to the public's beliefs, the public thus shares in jurisdiction-giving authority.

Understanding these four distinct task spaces as distinct jurisdictions with distinct audiences (or jurisdiction-givers) is key to understanding the source of the current crisis for the bioethics profession. The crisis is in public policy bioethics, spreading to cultural bioethics, and possibly eventually threatening health-care ethics consultation and research bioethics. Demarcating distinct jurisdictions is also key to understanding the resolution to the crisis for the bioethics profession, which is to shore up the health-care ethics consultation, research, and public policy bioethics jurisdictions by modifying the methods in the system of abstract knowledge so that they articulate better with the *new* views of the jurisdiction-givers, and to abandon competition for the cultural bioethics jurisdiction. Retreat from cultural bioethics is necessary because the bioethics profession has fallen prey to a well-recognized phenomenon in the professions where, as described in Abbott's canonical study of the professions, "as jurisdiction expands and as the ideas unifying it necessarily becomes more abstract, jurisdiction attenuates. . . . A profession already widely spread will . . . lose strength in its current jurisdictions if it claims yet another one, forcing its justifying abstractions to the limits of vagueness" (Abbott 1988:102, 104). It is time to retrench around the profession's strengths.

Bioethicists' Explanations of the Crisis in the Public Policy Bioethics Jurisdiction

We now need some more distinctions. There are two factions within the profession of bioethics, whom I will label the liberals and the conservatives. While these are not ideal titles, they comport with how most people see the debate. "Liberal" bioethicists would not have labeled themselves as such until the recent emergence of "conservative" bioethicists, as the liberals described their own views as neutral or universal. Indicative of their long-term dominance, liberals are also often called "mainstream" bioethicists.

In the view of liberal bioethicists, the emergent conservatives did not accept what bioethicist Jonathan Moreno calls "the Great Bioethics Compromise"—that technology is largely good, and should be encouraged with some guidance (Moreno 2005; Moreno and Berger 2010:xvii). Similarly, R. Alta Charo writes that there is "a cultural divide in the bioethics world that has been brewing for years. This divide, between those who celebrate the transformative power of science and those who fear it, is both broad and profound" (Charo 2004:311).

The "techno-skeptic" conservative group came to be publicly prominent with President George W. Bush's President's Council on Bioethics. Arthur Caplan acknowledges that "those on the left, secular end of bioethics had historically dominated most federal bodies . . . [but] with the appointment of Leon Kass to chair the President's Council, a new wind blew into Washington from the right. . . . Secular liberals stewed, fretted, and griped; conservatives and religious bioethicists offered support and praise" (Caplan 2005:12).

> On the one side is an alliance of neoconservative and religiously oriented bioethicists. They are wary of where biomedicine and biotechnology are taking us. They speak in terms that are religious or quasi-religious. They have established their own journals, think tanks, and training rograms. They operate in the corridors of power both in the White House and in Congress. They are at ease with the Republican party. They are backed by the deep pockets of very conservative foundations and wealthy philanthropists. They have no hesitance in saying that they operate as bioethicists.

> On the other side stand a loose amalgam of left-liberal bioethicists tenuously allied with a far smaller number of more libertarian bioethicists. This group is, on the whole, more at ease with the Democratic party. They are also more at ease with science and technology than their conservative counterparts. While not always in love with every thought, proposal, experiment, or initiative emanating from the world of bioscience and technology, they have no inherent fear or loathing of a scientific worldview. Indeed, they place their bets for a better tomorrow on scientific and technological progress. They speak primarily in secular terms drawn more from philosophy or the law. Explicitly religious arguments

get them nervous. They tend to dominate academia and the major bioethics programs located there (Caplan 2005:12).

The two sides have a high wall between them. Indeed, William May, a member of the bioethics commission of the George W. Bush era, describes bioethics as "a field that had broken up into a series of Balkan states, clearly not so dismembered as old Yugoslavia but nevertheless a contested terrain" (May 2010:257).

In the view of liberal bioethicists, the crisis is the result of the incivility between the two factions that makes people not want to listen to the profession (Macklin 2010). For example, Caplan writes that it is "the level of emotion characteristic of many current debates" that may "simply disqualify bioethics and bioethicists from their historic and hard-earned role as independent voices of reason, as well as trustworthy sources of objective analysis in an America still deeply divided along religious, cultural, class, ethnic, and racial lines" (Caplan 2005:13). Similarly, in his article decrying the demise of the Great Bioethics Compromise—the position in favor of techno-enthusiasm—Moreno writes that bioethics grew

> partly because it promised to provide a space for morally neutral, apolitical discourse. Within the field, the Compromise allowed its members to participate in this understanding. For many reasons, including the charged environment created by a deeply divided policy, the event of the President's Council of Bioethics has occasioned a shock to the field's academic civility and a consequent threat to the Great Bioethics Compromise (Moreno 2005:21).

The crisis, in this view, is caused by two sides that cannot reach agreement, not allowing the profession of bioethics to speak with an authoritative voice.

My Explanation of the Crisis in the Public Policy Bioethics Jurisdiction

While bioethicists tend to see the rise of conservative bioethics as the cause of the crisis, I see that as a recent symptom of a much more long-term disease, and we must treat the disease, not the symptoms. To solve the actual crisis, we must ask what allowed the formation of liberal and conservative factions in the first place. The deep cause is the delegitimation of the methods in the system of abstract knowledge of the bioethics profession. This in turn allowed for two events; one, the rise of a divided bioethics profession; two, the growth of the true competitor for jurisdiction with the bioethics profession—social-movement activists.

Liberal bioethicists like Caplan see their competitor as the conservatives. I see it differently, with both groups being part of the bioethics profession as they are both using the same system of abstract knowledge (albeit using different methods). The actual competitor with bioethics in public policy and cultural bioethics is social-movement activists, and both the liberals and the conservatives will be pushed aside with the continued growth of the activists' jurisdictional challenge. I do not consider social-movement activists to fit the sociological definition of a profession, so I will simply call them a group trying to take away jurisdiction from the bioethicists. This would then be both taking away of jurisdiction and "de-professionalization," but no matter—what is important for my purposes is that the task in the task space would not be conducted by bioethicists.

If the task in public policy bioethics is to provide ethical advice, the head of the National Right to Life Committee will do this for any government official or politician. The head of Planned Parenthood will do the same. The two social movements will provide advice to our elected officials, and as I will demonstrate in later chapters, it is these movements that increasingly control what actually happens on the most prominent bioethical issues in the US. Bioethicists can be upset that the advice given by the activists to elected officials concerning the end-of-life issues of the Terri Schiavo case was wrong, but bioethicists' suggestions were studiously ignored when it came to policy. The bioethics profession had de-legitimated itself, and the social movements are moving in to take over the jurisdictional space. The question then is: Why was the bioethics profession so vulnerable to this jurisdictional challenge? The rise of the social-movement activists as challengers goes back decades, and this rise itself—as well as the emergence of conservative bioethicists—is due to the delegitimation of the methods in the system of abstract knowledge of the bioethics profession.

The methods used in the system of abstract knowledge of the profession have been losing credibility for decades in the public policy bioethics task space because the views of the jurisdiction-giver have changed. Jurisdiction in public policy bioethics has traditionally been awarded by the government decision-makers such as officials at the National Institutes of Health who were the primary consumers of the ethical product. Unelected officials are strongly influenced by elected officials—when the elected officials care about the issue because they are being pressured by their constituents.

When the jurisdiction was originally forged, government officials were convinced by the bioethicists' methods. However, the politically active public that could influence elected officials, and thus unelected officials, began to change thirty years ago, in the early 1980s. Conservative religious people emerged as a force in the public sphere, and they do not accept that the bioethics profession is advocating for the general public's values in the public policy bioethics jurisdiction. They have let this view be known to elected policymakers and offer their own ethical analysis through their social movement generally known as the "religious right."

This is the cause of the crisis where the bioethics profession has less credibility, but the recently emerging symptom of competing factions within the profession has accelerated the disease. The presence of two competing factions in the bioethics profession itself de-legitimated the methods in the system of abstract knowledge of the bioethics profession due to the particular features of this system. It is not incivility per se that is the problem. Rather, merely having a contrary group within the profession demonstrates that the bioethics profession's methods do not produce the neutral ethics their system of abstract knowledge requires. The group bringing the greatest attention to this lack of neutrality was ironically the liberal bioethicists, who loudly bemoaned the influence of the new conservative group who did not share their values.

Indeed, in some statements, liberal bioethicists do not seem to even realize that they are undermining the legitimacy of their system of abstract knowledge by advertising that they are advocating a particular morality while claiming universality. Bioethicist Ruth Macklin, after seeming to identify the divide between the two groups in terms of the form of argument, basic notions of civility, and so on, gets in the last paragraph to the difference in values that underlie the two groups, writing that "[a]s a liberal, humanitarian bioethicist, I acknowledge that my chief concerns lie in striving for greater social justice within and among societies, and reducing disparities in health, wealth, and other resources among populations in the world. Unless the conservative bioethicists begin to address those topics, I for one will not find common cause with their main worries about where we are headed" (Macklin 2006:42). In other words, her values are from a subgroup of the population, and different from conservative citizens', and this admission advertises that the bioethicists' methods do not reflect the universal values of the public.

Some bioethicists *have* started to note that the claim that the bioethicists' methods lead to value neutrality is increasingly seen as untenable. Daniel Callahan, one of the founders of bioethical debate, criticized the liberal bioethicists' crisis containment strategy of more loudly proclaiming neutrality while claiming the conservatives are not neutral. He wrote:

> Why was it, for instance, that critics of Leon Kass's President's Council on Bioethics attacked its conservative cast as an

outrageous imposition of right-wing ideology on what should be a neutral body of rational deliberation—but failed to either note, or mention, that the three previous national commissions originated with Democratic administrations and featured liberal chairmen, liberal directors, liberal staffs, and overwhelmingly liberal members? Or failed to note that, in its deliberations and reports, there was far more internal division and dissent among the President's Council members than marked most of the other commissions? Kass's conservatism was out there on the surface, but its critics masked their underlying ideological bias (Callahan 2006:3).

Pellegrino similarly writes of the "diminishing confidence" with which "the public seeks assistance" of the "bioethics community" due to multiple opinions (Pellegrino 2006:576):

The strident and ever more virulent controversies within the bioethics community are damaging to bioethics and the public's confidence in bioethicists. In the face of issues of the gravest importance the public is confused. Many doubt there can be expert knowledge underlying such diversity of opinion. The public concludes that where there are so many opinions, there must not be any true opinion (Pellegrino 2006:578).

Callahan also sees that the exposure of the conflict in one jurisdiction will threaten all of the jurisdictions. Pointing to both the conservatives and the liberals ignoring each other, he writes that "the general public, and the medical and health policy world, will find it all too easy to dismiss bioethics as ideology driven, left or right politics in sheep's clothing. If we besmirch each other long enough, the public will soon conclude that we are all frauds" (Callahan 2005:431). That is, the conflict reveals that the methods used by the bioethics profession do not produce neutral ethics based

on the values of the entire population. To date, no one on the liberal bioethics side has called for examination of the methods in the
profession. They have, in my opinion, either simply hoped that the
conservatives would go away, or have moved toward becoming
social-movement activists who would represent only the liberal
subgroup of society.

Actually, the dean of the liberal wing of the profession, Arthur
Caplan, has come closest to accurately diagnosing the cause of the
crisis. In 2010 he wrote that:

> For at least two decades the field of bioethics has been at
> the center of the ideologically driven culture wars. As the
> right-to-life movement gained in organization and power
> in the Reagan, Bush One, and Bush Two administrations,
> both at the federal and state levels, many issues central to
> the bioethical canon—abortion, end-of-life care, assisted
> suicide, contraception, access to infertility services, disabil-
> ity rights, the care of newborns, organ donation, and the use
> of enhancement technologies—became defining issues for
> both the right and the left. Discontent with secular bioethics
> has led to the creation of think tanks and university pro-
> grams with explicit ties to evangelical Christianity or neo-
> conservative institutions. . . . The older image of a bioethics
> that stood neutral as a field while individual scholars took
> particular points of view is yielding to a world of politicized
> think tanks, commissions, advisory panels, councils, and
> foundations . . . it is fair to say that the fights of the past two
> decades are likely to ensure that the older model of purity
> will not be returning anytime soon (Caplan 2010:219).

But, like all bioethicists, he falls short and offers no solution to
the fact that conservatives have "discontent with secular bioethics"
and therefore the field does not produce neutral ethics. At the very
end of his essay he suggests that perhaps bioethicists will have to

"operate from explicit ideological perspectives." That is, they would implicitly give up on the claim to represent everyone, and join the ranks of social-movement activists, which would eliminate the profession as it has typically been defined. He does not discuss the problems that would cause. He then cryptically says "there may be other ways," but offers no solutions (Caplan 2010:223). I think claims to speak for everyone's ethics can be salvaged, and I offer one way out of the crisis in this book.

If the bioethics profession were to follow Caplan's suggestion and give up its system of abstract knowledge where it claims to be representing the values of individuals facing a decision or the general public it would lose its jurisdiction over both health-care ethics consultation and research bioethics. Were it to abandon its system of abstract knowledge it also would—and should, in my opinion— lose its jurisdiction over public policy bioethics. In the public policy bioethics task space, without the claim to be representing the public's morality, public policy bioethics becomes another spoil of the political system, indistinguishable from the social movements challenging for jurisdiction. In this case, the social group that wins at the polls recommends only its own ethics for public law. Those whose values are not represented by the party in power are frozen out. Indeed, this is where we are headed now, as the claims of bioethicists are coming to be seen as simply the ethics of one political faction.

So, in sum, the bioethics profession has traditionally legitimated its multiple jurisdictions in the public sphere by using a system of abstract knowledge wherein the profession is a neutral arbiter of others' values. The emergence of a conservative faction and social-movement activists are late-stage symptoms of a decades-long deterioration of the claim that the bioethicists' methods result in the representation of the entire public's values. This has created a crisis for the bioethics profession in, certainly, the public policy bioethics jurisdiction, and to a lesser extent for the cultural bioethics jurisdiction. There is a good-sized segment of the public and political elites

who are willing to just ignore bioethicists and turn to social movements for ethical advice on bioethical issues.

Solving the Bioethics Profession's Jurisdictional Crisis

Some may say that bioethics debates should be partisan and driven
by social-movement activists—and that we should decide the policy
of these issues through our elected officials. If the public concludes
that they want to ban embryonic stem cell research, they should just
vote Republican; if they support it, they should vote Democratic.
This will make the most sense to those who have extreme views on
bioethical issues, who see no value whatsoever in their views of their
adversaries. One might put the advocates of almost total libertarianism in embryo policy in this camp with the conservative Catholic
who believes that all manipulation of embryos—and certainly their
death—is always wrong. These are the people who influence the
positions of the political parties through social movements, as it is
the party activists who are the most extreme. For everyone else,
communicative institutions that reach across differences are helpful. Many of the bioethical issues are so novel that to eliminate
a priori any ideas about it would damage our ability to deal with the
issue. We need debates across differences, and bioethical debate
facilitates this. The profession of bioethics can serve a particularly
useful role.

   To solve the crisis in the public policy bioethics jurisdiction,
I advocate retaining the system of abstract knowledge wherein
bioethical claims represent the values of participants in the ethical
decision (health-care ethics consultation) or of the general public
(research bioethics; public policy bioethics). I advocate for new
methods so that ethical recommendations *are* representing the
claims of others.

Summary of Future Chapters

In the first section of this book, I will describe the emergence of bioethical debates, the historical differentiation of the four task spaces, and the rise of the profession of bioethics. Particular social forces caused these developments, and we must keep these forces in mind when advocating solutions to the crisis. In the second section of book, I will delve deeper into the source of the crisis for the profession of bioethics; and in the final section, I will describe reforms that would create methods in the system of abstract knowledge that will be more legitimate in the jurisdictions bioethics claims.

I break down the history of bioethical debate into three eras, starting in the early 1960s. In the first, scientists and physicians had solid, almost unquestioned jurisdiction over health-care ethics consultation and research bioethics. Scientists also began to seek jurisdiction over a task long implicitly controlled by the theological profession—cultural ethical debate about the purpose of technology and medicine. The theologians quickly realized that their jurisdiction was under threat, and fought back, using the theological discourse and methods that comprised *their* system of abstract knowledge.

Quickly realizing the hopelessness of defeating this challenge from scientists while using their established system of abstract knowledge, in the second era the theologians began to make exclusively secular arguments in their attempt to defend their jurisdiction. This was more suited for public debate in a religiously pluralistic society, and was, ironically, the predecessor to the methods used by bioethicists that would eventually defeat theology. Critically for the history of these debates, the theologians (with others) succeeded in getting the public concerned about ethical issues in science and medicine, and the public appealed to their government representatives for protection. The health-care ethics consultation and research bioethics jurisdictions held by science/medicine were now also threatened.

In the third era (described in Chapter 2), at the urging of theologians and other challengers, the government inserted itself as the jurisdiction-giver for a new task—providing ethical advice on biomedical policy matters (the public policy bioethics task space.) The government also replaced the public as the jurisdiction-giver in the health-care ethics consultation and research bioethics task spaces.

The new jurisdiction-givers, government officials, had different standards for how the tasks should be performed than the public did, which destabilized the entire professional competition for jurisdiction over these tasks. A new system of abstract knowledge was created that fit the interests of the new jurisdiction-givers, and this system ultimately defined the new bioethics profession. The system of abstract knowledge (and its profession of bioethics) very quickly established a very secure jurisdiction over health-care ethics consultation and research bioethics. It more slowly and more contentiously established a fairly strong jurisdiction over public policy bioethics and began to fight for jurisdiction over cultural bioethics. The system of abstract knowledge used by the theology profession was not a good fit with the new jurisdiction-givers, and theologians faded away, ironically defeated by the forces they first unleashed.

In the second section of the book I examine the emergence of the jurisdictional crisis of the bioethics profession. In Chapter 3, I describe the changing views of the jurisdiction-givers in the public policy bioethics jurisdiction. The emergent religious right in American politics, acting through the Republican Party, forced the jurisdiction-givers in the government to consider the religious right's values. These social-movement activists would not only give their own ethical advice, but they repeatedly demonstrated that the ethics of the commissions in the public policy bioethics jurisdiction were not neutral, resulting in a serious problem for the legitimacy claims of the bioethics profession. The government bioethics commission of President George W. Bush attempted to reformulate the methods of the bioethics profession to avoid the mechanisms that had worked against the inclusion of the conservatives' views. This in turn revealed a deep chasm in moral understanding among bioethicists. The common morality articulated by the liberal wing of the bioethics profession does not seem to be held by these conservatives, throwing into question how "common" this morality actually is.

In the final section of the book, I advocate for a fourth era of bioethical debate that has more secure jurisdictions for the bioethics profession. In Chapter 4, I complicate the historical narrative by showing that when bioethics replaced theology as the challenger to science/medicine, it actually accepted less-powerful jurisdictional relationships with the science/medicine profession. This arrangement meant that, while the profession could fulfill this role in the first two jurisdictions, it had difficulty with legitimacy in public policy bioethics.

The jurisdiction over health-care ethics consultation and research bioethics remains solid. In Chapter 5, I recommend solidifying jurisdiction over public policy bioethics by modifying the methods used in the system of abstract knowledge of the bioethics profession to make them more legitimate to the jurisdiction-givers. I advocate creating a modified version of common morality principlism where the common morality is empirically determined for each issue that is subject to health-care ethics consultation, research bioethics, and public policy bioethics. This retains the democratic legitimacy of the system of abstract knowledge used by bioethicists and retains the structural features that make it appealing to policy makers, while increasing the likelihood that providers of jurisdiction will really see it as representing the common morality. It will also eliminate a critique of conservatives, which is that under the guise of neutrality, the bioethics profession is simply advancing an ideology of the liberal professionals, the ideology of science, or the morality of the Democratic Party. It will simultaneously remove the analogous critique of liberals, that conservatives are similarly advancing a religious, conservative agenda. The methods in the system of abstract knowledge of the bioethics profession used for health-care ethics consultation and research bioethics then simply become specifications of this more general system. Participation in cultural bioethics by bioethicists would end, and I advocate that bioethicists who want to influence cultural bioethics should revert to another professional status that most have, such as "philosopher."

My advocacy of improving the methods in the system of abstract knowledge used by bioethicists is not intended to besmirch the people who invented these methods. However, these methods spread from their original applications, became institutionalized, and are now ill-suited for additional jurisdictions. Like the human appendix, an unadaptive feature that evolved due to its fit with a previous environment, the methods are no longer adaptive. Yet they continue. The appendix continues to exist due to the slowness of evolution; the methods in the bioethics system of abstract knowledge continue because they have become institutionalized.

Notes

1. Dzur (2002:178). Dzur and I ultimately differ on the role of bioethics professionals in the public sphere.

2. In an earlier book, I wrote about a subset of debate I labeled "public bioethical debate" (Evans 2002:34). In this book I break "public bioethical debate" into public policy bioethics and cultural bioethics in order to make finer distinctions.

3. There are many institutions in the public sphere that are largely composed of academics who serve a similar function. For example, there is a widespread debate about what we should do about "the family." There are academics, of whom I am most familiar with the sociologists of the family, who debate amongst themselves what is really going on with families. They interact, directly and indirectly, with scholars who make normative arguments about what families *should* be like. These people all shape the public mind in the public sphere from the larger soapbox they are given, contributing editorials to newspapers,

testifying before Congress, serving on government commissions, and writing books and articles.

4. Rutenberg, Jim. "In health-care debate, bioethicist becomes a lightning rod for criticism." *New York Times*, August 25, 2009. P. A11.

5. MCT News Service. "VA booklet on end-of-life issues for vets defended by ethicists, experts." *San Diego Union Tribune*, September 3, 2009. P. A5.

6. MCT News Service. "VA booklet on end-of-life issues for vets defended by ethicists, experts." *San Diego Union Tribune*, September 3, 2009. P. A5.

7. "Response to the recent attacks on bioethicists." American Society for Bioethics and the Humanities. August 25, 2009.

8. "Response to the recent attacks on bioethicists." American Society for Bioethics and the Humanities. August 25, 2009.

9. This is a slightly more expansive definition of "a member of the bioethics profession" than I had used in my previous work, which was limited to examining a narrower range of jurisdictions (Evans 2002:37).

10. H. Tristram Engelhardt has spent decades criticizing the profession's system of abstract knowledge, and he writes that the bioethics profession claims "to offer a basis for a consensus grounded in a common, secularly available morality" (Engelhardt 2007:121). Elsewhere, he writes that bioethics is "a special secular tradition that attempts to frame answers in terms of no particular tradition, but rather in ways open to rational individuals as such. . . . Bioethics is developing as the lingua franca of a world concerned with health care, but not possessing a common ethical viewpoint" (Engelhardt 1986:5).

11. In the 2011 report of the American Society of Bioethics and the Humanities concerning the "core competencies" of health-care ethics consultation (HCEC), they write that "there is a general consensus in the field that 'ethics facilitation' is the best model for HCEC." In ethics facilitation "recommendations(s) made should comport with the bioethics literature, medical literature, other relevant scholarly literature, current professional and practice standards in the field of HCEC, statues, judicial opinions, and pertinent institutional polices. And second, the process of pursuing resolution should be respectful of all the parties involved and their interests. The knowledge, the skills and the facilitative strategies of the HCEC should improve the likelihood of building an ethically supportable consensus among stakeholders" (American Society for Bioethics and Humanities 2011:9). Note that the "bioethics

literature" in health-care ethics consultation is largely based on common morality principlism, and is thus also representing the values of the general public (see below). They explicitly reject the "authoritarian approach" wherein the ethics consultants use their own values to tell the parties what they should do.

12. Shalit, in Dzur (2002:195). As for bioethicists who claim that they have no moral expertise and claim no special authority, I agree with Carl Elliott that such a claim fails to comprehend that it is not what you claim, but the position you have been given that makes people assume you have expertise. "There is something disingenuous about a bioethicist who claims to have no special expertise yet happily occupies the seat of an expert on the television news" (Elliott 2007:45).

13. Beauchamp (1982:14). It is notable that Beauchamp, one of the founders and contemporary promoters of common-morality principlism, does not include the derivation of common moral principles as a bioethical skill.

14. Persad et al. (2008:89, 90). This study of teaching bioethics in medical school finds that 100% of medical schools associated with the Association of American Medical Colleges comply with this requirement, with an average of 35.6 hours of instruction.

15. The ethics commission that recommends policy is also often used by professionals in suggesting policy for industry trade groups (e.g., Biotechnology Industry Organization) or corporations (e.g., Advanced Cell Technology) (Brody et al. 2002). An ethical question here might be whether a corporation should engage in therapeutic cloning. Because any such policy would not be applied to all citizens, and would never be seen as representing the values of the public, it is not part of public policy bioethics as I have defined it. Professionals engaging in this would not be "bioethicists."

Commissions are also used to provide advice to the often quasi-governmental advice-providing intellectual institutions such as the Institutes of Medicine, National Academies, and the American Academy for the Advancement of Science. These sorts of entities often produce reports that are similar to those of government ethics commissions. To the extent that they are recommending policies to be implemented by the government, I will treat them like the governmental ethics commissions. To the extent that they are recommending what the public's ethics *should be* about a technology or practice, I will consider them to be institutions in cultural bioethics (see below).

16. Although I take this term from Callahan (1999:279), I use it somewhat differently than he does. Callahan also describes health policy bioethics, which I consider part of public policy bioethics, and foundational bioethics, which is essentially academic–meta theory about ethics and debates about the proper system of abstract knowledge of the bioethics profession.

17. Jensen conducted a study of one of the methods of using the system of abstract knowledge of the bioethics profession in media discourse about therapeutic cloning in the United States and the United Kingdom. He found that the system was dominant before 2000, but lost out from 2001 forward (Jensen 2008:196), which is consistent with the timing of the growing crisis I describe later.

PART I

The History of Bioethical Debate and the Bioethics Profession

Chapter 1

The Emergence of Bioethical Debate and the Jurisdictional Struggle Between Science and Theology

Medical ethics has an ancient history, which we can ignore for the purposes of this book. For our purposes we can start in the 1960s, and it is often quipped that what we think of as the "1960s"—with protests against establishments and the like—actually began in 1968. However, in discussions about the ethics of science and medicine the questioning of "the Establishment" actually *did* begin in 1960. The explosion in scientific research following World War II had begun to bear fruit, and scientists were now questioning its effects, as well as contemplating research that had before then been inconceivable.

Science was seen as producing a number of side-effects with momentous implications such as environmental pollution and over-population, which were seen as the results of improving agriculture and medicine. Technological improvements also suggested to scientists that humans would soon have a degree of control over themselves that had previously been the stuff of science fiction: mind control, human cloning, human genetic engineering, test-tube babies, parthenogenesis, human/animal chimeras, artificial organs and body parts, and the transplantation of more symbolic body parts (such as the heart), which had not been accomplished as the decade began. As many noted at the time, scientists would have to make distinctions that they had not had to worry about before, such as when someone is "really" dead so that their organs can be removed. The response from one participant in this debate typifies the response to all of these emergent technologies: "Man's existence now, and for the first time, is threatened" (Chisholm 1963:315).

During the 1960s, what bioethicist Albert Jonsen has called the "decade of conferences," scientists had many meetings to discuss the "Brave New World" that beckoned them. A conference in the early 1960s in London is a good example, and it brought together many leading scientists of the day, such as Sir Julian Huxley, Hermann Muller, Joshua Lederberg, and J. B. S. Haldane. The agenda was to discuss the genetic modification of humans, population control, the elimination of disease, and mind control. The conference proceedings, published under the telling title *Man and His Future*, noted in the preface that

> the world was unprepared socially, politically and ethically for the advent of nuclear power. Now, biological research is in a ferment, creating and promising methods of interference with "natural processes" which could destroy or could transform nearly every aspect of human life which we value. Urgently it is necessary for men and women . . . to consider the present and imminent possibilities (Wolstenholme 1963:v).

It was era of questioning ends, not just the means. "Where are we taking ourselves with our new technological abilities?" was the central theme. As the dean of the Dartmouth Medical School stated at the opening of perhaps the first of these conferences in 1960, "Although [medicine's] foundations have become more rational, its practice . . . is said to have become more remote and indifferent to human values, and once again medicine has been forced to remind itself that it is often the human factors that are determinant." The point of the conference was "not simply the question of the survival or the extinction of man, but *what kind* of survival? A future of what *nature*?" (Cited in Jonsen 1998:13). I consider these conversations to be the emergence of the cultural bioethics task space: public policy bioethics had not yet been created, and research bioethics and health-care ethics consultation were uncontestedly under the jurisdiction of scientists and physicians.

During these early years, scientists kept the cultural bioethics debate limited to scientists. They recognized that the topic of "where mankind should go" with new technology was, in the public mind, under the jurisdiction of the profession of theology, but many of the elite scientists were attempting a jurisdictional expansion into the jurisdiction held by theology. They thought that science should produce a sense of meaning and source of ethics for human society—given that, in their view, religion had been utterly discredited after Darwin. For example, C. H. Waddington and Peter Medawar would imply, along with other biologists, that "the 'direction' of evolution, both biological and cultural, is the 'scientific' foundation upon which to reestablish our system of ethics and to rest 'our most cherished hopes.' . . ." (Kaye 1997:42). Similarly, population geneticist Theodosius Dobzhansky believed that "restored to the 'Center of the Universe' by the wisdom and beneficence of evolution, man is free to seek beauty, justice, and self-transcendence and not 'mere survival'" (Kaye 1997:42).

Robert Edwards, the first scientist to engage in in-vitro fertilization, was also part of this expansionist project. In this autobiography he reflected on his views of science, referencing the key figures of this era. Edwards complained that "many non-scientists see a more limited role for science, almost a fact-gathering exercise providing neither values, morals, nor standards. . . . My answer . . . is that moral laws must be based on what man knows about himself, and that this knowledge inevitably comes largely from science." Given that science is the only legitimate way of knowing, Edwards references the ideas of physicist Jacob Bronowski and then concludes by agreeing with biologist Julian Huxley that "Today the God hypothesis has ceased to be scientifically tenable, has lost its explanatory value and is becoming an intellectual burden to our thought" (Edwards 1989:165–166).

The scientists were clear about who their primary competitor for jurisdiction was. As Bronowski would pronounce at one of these conferences in 1962: "I am, therefore, not in the least ashamed to be told by somebody else that my values, because they are grounded in my science, are relative, and his are given by God. My values, in my opinion, come from as objective and definitive a source as any god, namely the nature of the human being. . . . That makes my values richer, I think; and it makes them no less objective, no less real, than any values that can be read in the Testaments" (Wolstenholme 1963:372). The first pull-quote on the back cover of the published conference proceedings was from Francis Crick, co-discoverer of the structure of DNA, who agreed, writing, "I think that in time the facts of science are going to make us become less Christian. There is eventually bound to be a conflict of values." In short, science was in a triumphalist mode, and could try to take over tasks long under the jurisdiction of the theology profession.

In response, theologians engaged in an attempt to fight off these professional interlopers, a defense to counteract the long line of jurisdictions that had been taken from them by other professions, as extensively described in the literature on secularization (Smith 2003). I will chart three short eras in the time between the initial efforts of scientists to gain jurisdiction over emerging bioethical debates and the surrender of the theological profession.

Many observers have discussed this period of time coinciding with the theological retreat, albeit with less detail. For example, M. Therese Lysaught describes the "standard narrative of the genesis of bioethics," saying "its earliest origins lay among theologians, but substantive theological discourse was quickly replaced by the more advanced discourse of philosophy" (Lysaught 2006:101). Albert Jonsen similarly portrays the common wisdom among bioethics professionals as "bioethics began in religion, but religion has faded from bioethics" (Jonsen 2006:23). The decline of theologians in these debates is not disputed (Evans 2002; Cahill 2005; Jonsen 2006; Childress 2003; Messikomer, Fox and Swazey 2001; Callahan 1990;

Lammers 1996; Marty 1992; Walters 1985; Engelhardt 1986:5). What is not as often analyzed is why this decline occurred, and what it means for the present state of bioethical debate.

The standard argument for the defeat of the theologians by the bioethicists is that society began to demand recognition of pluralism in the 1960s. Engelhardt summarizes this view well, and is worth quoting at length:

> The history of bioethics over the last two decades has been the story of the development of a secular ethic. Initially, individuals working from within particular religious traditions held the center of bioethical discussions. However, this focus was replaced by analyses that span traditions, including particular secular traditions. As a result, a special secular tradition that attempts to frame answers in terms of no particular tradition, but rather in ways open to rational individuals as such, has emerged. Bioethics is an element of a secular culture and the great-grandchild of the Enlightenment. . . . That is, the existence of open, peaceable discussion among divergent groups, such as atheists, Catholics, Jews, Protestants, Marxists, heterosexuals and homosexuals, about public policy issues bearing on health care, will press unavoidably for a neutral common language. Bioethics is developing as the lingua franca of a world concerned with health care, but not possessing a common ethical viewpoint (Engelhardt 1986:5).

I think that this standard narrative about the defeat of theology is but one part of the story, and to understand the challenges facing bioethics today, we must provide a more detailed explanation.

An important distinction between these eras in my history of bioethical debate is in the nature of the arguments that theologians made. I analyze these arguments as concerning means and ends, and an "end" is the value or goal being forwarded. For example, many arguments in bioethical debate are explicitly or implicitly forwarding the end of improving health. The means are actions—in our case, typically, biomedical technologies—that may be consistent with or maximize the ends one is implicitly or explicitly advocating. For example, a typical argument is that somatic cell human genetic engineering (a means) is ethically acceptable because it is advancing the healing of disease (an end).

With these terms in mind, in the first era, theologians made arguments that had secular ends that were explicit, condensed translations of theological ends. A condensed translation takes a very elaborated, detailed end and creates a simplified, less precise and more general end. Through generalization it was hoped that the new end would match a condensed translation of some other group's elaborate, detailed end. Thus, Protestants and Catholics could agree on an end to pursue in human experimentation or genetic engineering without having to agree on the details. Part of generalization is abandoning the explicitly theological language. The key is that these condensed translations are unbiased—they are less precise and more general, but they still accurately portray the core of the value or end being pursued.

Later, I will distinguish a condensed translation from a transmutation, which takes a part of the original end or value that fits with an established end or value, even if the part is not central to the original end, while nonetheless claiming that the original end or value is represented by the transmutation. For example, pieces of Catholic theology can be made to fit with Protestant theology, but only by taking peripheral elements from each Catholic idea that happen to fit with Protestantism. Catholics would not consider this an accurate *translation*, but a *transmutation*.[1]

In a contemporary condensed translation, a theologian could conclude that as we are all created in the image of God, technological means should respect the sacredness of each person. This could be condensed and translated to the secular end of pursuing the Kantian "respect for persons." Theologians were then not arguing about the theology itself, but were arguing about the various ends that they thought should be relevant for medicine and science. This era was short-lived, and many scholars do not recognize that it existed at all.[2]

The second era began with the rapid retreat by theologians who gave up on *explicitly* translating theological ends, and fell back into having the ethics of science and medicine focus on secularly stated ends that were *implicit* condensed translations of theological ends. However, the theologians in this second era were conflicted. While some continued with the implicit condensed translation method, and tried to persuade the public to accept these ends, others began to search for ends that were already universally held by all people, regardless of their theological persuasion. This seed planted by a faction of the theologians ironically grew into a challenge to the jurisdiction of theology when this seed grew into the system of abstract knowledge of the new profession of bioethics. The bioethics profession did not begin with theological ends and translate to secular language, thus resulting in a debate about various ends. Rather it started with a list of four ends portrayed as the values held by all of the citizens, which one could transmute other ends into. As bioethicists gained strength, the theological challenge slowly receded, and it was the bioethicists who would wrest jurisdiction from the scientists.

These three eras occurred in such rapid succession that it difficult to consider them separately. Indeed there is substantial overlap— even in the earliest era of explicit theological ends the first theologians searching for secular universal ends were beginning to write. Even in the final era there remained some unrepentant theologians arguing for condensed translations of explicitly theological ends. The three eras are like three bell-shaped curves on an axis with a high degree of overlap, revealing three distinct peaks, but with the majority of the area under the curve coinciding with the one next to it. In this chapter I will examine the first two distinct peaks, and in the next chapter the third, while simply acknowledging the more complicated picture that lies in the overlapping tails of the curves.

Excursus on Religion in the United States

It is well known, yet rarely acknowledged, that all of these first theologians in cultural bioethical debate would be, by today's standards, religious liberals and not religious conservatives.[3] And, as my narrative develops in subsequent chapters, I will show that the later increase in religious voices in debates about bioethical issues is from conservative, not liberal religious voices. Therefore, a basic understanding of American religion is critical.

Skipping from the voyage of the Mayflower in 1620 three hundred years forward, in the 1920s Protestantism dominated public life in the United States. Yes, there were religious minorities like Jews, Mormons, and others, but their influence on public life was even less than would be expected given their numbers. There were increasing numbers of Roman Catholics, but they were largely the despised immigrants of their day, and were not integrated into positions of power in the public sphere but rather a religion that the Protestant elite thought it needed to control.

In the 1920s there was a "culture war" within Protestantism between the modernists and the fundamentalists (Noll 1992:Ch. 14). They clashed over many issues, but as an example, consider biblical interpretation. A modernist could show, using modern literary methods, that if you go back to the original Hebrew, the prophet Isaiah was not prophesizing that a "virgin" would bear a son, but that a "young woman" would bear a son. What is more familiar to most people is the willingness of the modernists to engage with the materialist science at the time, particularly Darwinism and geology, to say that the traditional Genesis narrative is not literally true. Fundamentalists were, generally, biblical literalists, fairly separatist, and socially conservative. The modernists had more social power: they were the heads of colleges, the professionals, the elected officials, the journalists, and so on. The theological descendants of the modernists are now called "mainline Protestants." And, to get a bit ahead of myself, these mainline Protestants are the people who in the 1960s were prominent in the theological response to the jurisdictional challenge from science.

It is hard to summarize mainline Protestantism in a paragraph, but to give you a sense of its orientation, mainliners are not biblical literalists. A classic mainline phrase would be: "the Bible was written by people struggling to understand God." Second, mainliners are socially more liberal than other Protestants. For example, their denominations defended the *Roe v. Wade* abortion decision for many years; they are the denominations most likely to ordain women; and they are the denominations currently having the debate about gay marriages and gay clergy. They are, to put it quite simply, "more liberal" than other Protestants.

Organizationally, while people of a mainline theological orientation could exist in many denominations, they are concentrated in a number of denominations dominant between the colonial era and the 1960s. For example, the United Church of Christ, the Episcopal Church, the United Methodist Church, the Presbyterian Church (USA), the Evangelical Lutheran Church in America, and the American Baptist Churches would all be considered generally mainline. The most liberal of these, the United Church of Christ, was massively overrepresented among the early theological voices in bioethical debate.

The fundamentalist–modernist split was roughly centered in the 1920s. In the 1940s there was another split, this time within fundamentalism. For readers who are not from this conservative Protestant world, this may seem like splitting hairs, but a group of people, the most famous of whom was the Reverend Billy Graham, thought that the fundamentalists were too rigid and the modernists too wishy-washy. They created a new movement called "evangelicalism" as a halfway stop between fundamentalism and mainline Protestantism. Evangelicals could be thought of as liberal fundamentalists or conservative mainline Protestants. Taking some more contemporary exemplars, the Reverend Jerry Falwell was a fundamentalist, and former president George W. Bush is an evangelical. Again, these may seem like small distinctions if one is not from this world, but evangelicals are more liberal than fundamentalists on theological matters, like biblical interpretation. They are also much less separatist, and are actively engaged in the world. Both fundamentalists and evangelicals are, in my terms, conservative Protestants.

Again, while evangelicals exist in many Protestant denominations, they are concentrated in a number of denominations such as the Southern Baptist Churches, the Church of the Nazarene, the Presbyterian Church in America, the Assemblies of God, the Christian Reformed Church, and many more. Fundamentalists eschew denominations, and tend to not believe in organization above the congregational level, with most of those congregations calling themselves Baptist.

A critical point for the development of bioethical debate is that *both* the fundamentalists and the evangelicals took one lesson from their split with the modernists in the 1920s; which was that the mainline establishment was opposed to them, and that they should retreat from national public life and focus on saving souls. Mainline Protestantism continued to be the one religion to dominate the public sphere up until the 1960s or 1970s. In the 1960s, lessened discrimination against Catholics and Jews meant that these groups were slowly allowed into the conversation, but only to the extent that their form of argumentation was similar to the way that mainline Protestants made their arguments. Much has been said about the Protestantization of Catholicism, but let us just say that it was the more liberal Catholics who were a part of the theological group defending jurisdiction—those whose thinking about these issues most closely emulated that of the mainline Protestants. But, even in the 1960s and 1970s, fundamentalists and evangelicals largely remained aloof from the public sphere, at least on medical or scientific issues, despite their fairly large numbers in terms of the overall population of the United States.

In the Beginning: Condensed Translation of Explicitly Theological Ends

Returning to our discussion of the first era, the scientists in the early 1960s were triumphant after their success in WWII and the 1950s. They were seemingly poised to engage in novel experiments such as merging two forms of life by merging their DNA, suggesting that the new scientific vision could be used to shape humans themselves. A faction of scientists had been engaged in an attempt to take away the jurisdiction of theologians over explaining the meaning and purpose of humanity, which was seemingly at stake in these technological developments. Some scientists, perhaps not believing that scientists had an answer for everything, urged that the public be consulted. For scientists to "claim the right to decide alone" about the direction of scientific efforts, said viral geneticist Salvador Luria, would be "to advocate technocracy" (Luria 1965:3, 17). By mid-decade, according to historian of science Susan Wright, "growing numbers of people—including many scientists—began finding the social role and impact of modern science and technology increasingly problematic. . . . Public confidence in technological development as the key to social progress gave way to disenchantment" (Wright 1994:36–37). Scientists would not be able to simply gain jurisdiction through assertion, but would have to debate with theology to make their case.

Given how much ground theology had lost in public life in previous decades, one has to wonder why they bothered to resist the challenge of scientists for jurisdiction over cultural bioethics. One reason may have been that theologians saw that their remaining jurisdiction of helping *individuals* determine the meaning and purpose of life was also threatened by the scientists' jurisdictional challenge. For example, Methodist theologian and Princeton religion professor Paul Ramsey (1913–1988) recognized that the scientists posed a challenge to theology's core jurisdiction.[4] Ramsey was not simply opposed to some of the emerging technologies, but was actually opposed to what he called a "surrogate theology" of the "cult" of "messianic positivism" led by scientists. At a 1965 conference, he used the phrase "playing God" to summarize the form of argumentation used by the scientists—what he called their "worldview"—saying that the scientists' goal was to provide the meaning of life:

> ... taken as a whole, the proposals of the revolutionary biologists, the anatomy of their basic thought-forms, the ultimate context for acting on these proposals provides a propitious place for learning the meaning of "playing God"— in contrast to being men on earth.
>
> [The scientists have] "a distinctive attitude toward the world," "a program for utterly transforming it," an "unshakable," nay even a "fanatical," confidence in a "worldview," a "faith" no less than a "program" for the reconstruction of mankind. These expressions rather exactly describe a religious cult, if there ever was one—a cult of men-gods, however otherwise humble. These are not the findings, or the projections, of an exact science as such, but a religious view of where and how ultimate human significance is to be found. It is a proposal concerning mankind's final hope. One is reminded of the words of Martin Luther to the effect that we have either God or an idol and "whatever your heart trusts in and relies on, that is properly your God" (Ramsey 1970a:143–144).

There were many other conferences and controversies in science and medicine where theologians challenged scientists. Consider, for example, the conference that was held in reaction to the first heart transplant in 1967. This conference was to address the "clinical, moral, ethical, theological and psychological implications" of this technology, and despite the supposed range of topics, three of the six speakers were theologians (and one more was Jesuit Robert Drinan, a Catholic legal scholar). While not as explicit as Ramsey in naming the scientific opponent, German theologian Helmut Thielicke, in discussing the ethics of deciding who should get a transplant, given the limited supply, provided an explicit condensed translation of theological ideas into the secular end of "infinite worth":

> One possibility is to understand the value and dignity of man in terms of his "utility," for example, his capacity to function in the productive process, or his biological or historical potential. . . . The physician, for example, has to realize that in adopting this view of man he surrenders his healing ethos and becomes an engineer, a technician doing manipulations for a productive society. . . . There is an alternative, however, to this view of man in terms of his "utility." One can speak instead of his "infinite worth," a worth over which I have no control. And here I must say quite openly that I know of no place in the world where the inviolability of man is so expressly attested and defended as in the Bible. . . . The basis of human dignity is seen to reside not in any immanent quality of man whatsoever, but in the fact that God created him. Man is the apple of God's eye. He is "dear" because he has been bought with a price: Christ died for him (Thielicke 1970:169–170).

In sum, he was arguing that we should adopt as an end the idea of each human's "infinite worth," which is a translation of the theological end defined by the Crucifixion.

Counter-attacking the scientists was plausible because theology had a well-developed discourse to address the purpose of science and medicine. Catholicism had a very long history of explicitly Catholic medical ethics, and Protestants, while not having the same depth, nonetheless had a long tradition of discourse about suffering, the body, and the purpose of human life. These early theologians knew that not all of the hearers of their claims would share their explicitly theological premises, but seemed to feel that Christian theology was widely enough shared and dominant that it could be accepted.

Ramsey seemed to insist on the theological basis for his work before translating. While acknowledging that not all were Christians, he seemed to be writing for that group he assumed were still within the orbit of Christian belief, and urging them to come back into the fold.[5] For example, in discussing the ethics of the giving of vital organs, in 1969, Ramsey's reasoning would include the following:

> From the standpoint of Christian ethics within the tradition of the Reformation, however, charity (*agape*) is a free act of grace—first in God's gift of himself in love to man, and then in man's gift of himself in love to neighbor. . . .
>
> It is, therefore, important to mention a "counter argument" within the structure of Protestant ethics insofar as this has been more profoundly Biblical than past Catholic moralists. Biblical authors not only speak of love to God and Neighbor. They also hold a very realistic view of the life of man who is altogether flesh (*sarx*). God is in heaven, man is on earth. . . . No one who has been consciously formed by Biblical perspectives is likely to be beguiled by notions of the person whose origin actually is a Cartesian dualism of mind and body; nor will he yield to the enchantment of mystical, spiritual notions of unearthly communion with God and fellow man. . . .
>
> From this point of view, one must ask of any Christian, who today without any hesitation flies into the wild blue yonder of transcendent human spiritual achievement while submitting the body unlimitedly to medical and other technologies, whether his outlook is not rather a product of Cartesian mentalism and dualism, and one that, for all its religious and personalistic terminology, has no longer any Biblical comprehension of joy in creaturely life and the acceptable death of all who are flesh (Ramsey 1970b:185–188).

Here we have fairly explicit theology translated into secular ends. As in much of his work, he is writing for that scientist or physician who, if not still Christian, had perhaps attended church as a child—those who have "been consciously formed by Biblical perspectives." He did think his secularly stated ends should be broadly comprehensible.

In 1970, Ramsey published a book titled *The Patient as Person* that is his most influential secular condensed translation of a theological end. According to theologian M. Therese Lysaught, in the text Ramsey starts with "the scriptural narrative of God's covenant with the people of Israel and eventually all of humanity." This covenant means that "God—transcendent beyond all knowing—promises fidelity, care, presence, and sustenance to creatures vastly unequal to the divine being" (Lysaught 2004:672). These values were translated into the secular (and Kantian) concept of "respect for persons." Lysaught continues: "Being a theologian, Ramsey had no qualms about fleshing out his Kantian sensibilities in theological terms," drawing in this book and elsewhere on theologian Karl Barth (Lysaught 2004:673). One implication of "respect for persons" is that scientists had to ask the permission of people they were going to experiment upon, as "informed consent is 'expressive of the respect for the man who is the subject in medical investigations'" (Lysaught 2004:673). According to another analyst of Ramsey's career, Ramsey made use of consent because he "sought to find a language accessible to as many people as possible despite their theological convictions and 'consent' appeared to cross over communities and traditions" (Long 1993:125–126). This is the epitome of the motivation for a condensed translation.

Ramsey was on the more conservative end of the theologians who engaged in the jurisdictional counter-attack on science. Although later scholars of this era have wondered why Ramsey became involved in the confrontation with science and medicine (Walters 1985), after writing extensively on topics such as peace and war, it seemed he was partially provoked by his long-term sparring partner in theological debates—Joseph Fletcher—whom Ramsey saw as implicitly promoting the jurisdictional expansion of the scientists.

Fletcher was probably the first American Protestant to enter debates about the ethics of medicine in modern times, writing a book in 1954 that was essentially an attempt to create a Protestant medical ethics in reaction to the long-standing Catholic medical ethics (Fletcher 1993). This was still a time when mainline Protestant theologians thought that they were the religious representatives of our culture, and that all good professionals fit into the Protestant-Catholic-Jew model of the 1950s articulated by Herberg. "Every doctor has loyalty, we may assume, to certain medical ideals [and] loyalty to religious convictions . . ." begins the preface to Fletcher's book. It continues: "Dr. Fletcher has examined the ethical problems and the value systems of physicians, in the light of our Judaeo-Christian culture" (Fletcher 1954:vii–viii).

It was Fletcher's later role as the leading proponent of situation ethics, particularly in issues of medicine and science, that would arouse Ramsey's ire (Attwood 1992:29). The details of this debate between Fletcher and Ramsey are beyond the scope of this book, but suffice it to say they were arguing about how to translate the Christian end of *agape* in the world—either means should be consistent with this end through Ramsey's rules or the possible means should maximize *agape* free of rules, for Fletcher. The point is that they were both still forwarding explicitly Christian ends, translated into secular ends.

The Beginning of the Decline: Pluralism and Secular Ends

As much as I have tried to raise the explicitly Christian ends forwarded in the writings of the theologians, they were already shifting toward the second era. What took place was a move from condensed translation of *explicitly* theological ends to the use of only secular ends that were at best *implicit* translations of theological ends.

The general reason for this transition was, to put it colloquially, a heavy dose of realism as to how far the secularization of the public sphere had already progressed (Smith 2003). To put it differently, a little bit of experience revealed that the jurisdiction they were defending was incredibly weak. These new issues had been framed in the public as new issues that arose from scientific experimentation, but without an explicit form of ethics to connect to these new issues, the jurisdiction of the theologians was almost instinctual, as in "that sounds like a theological question." However, many public participants in these early debates did not think it obvious that these were theological questions and that theologians should have jurisdiction.

Consider a conference on "the sanctity of life" held in 1966 at Reed College. The organizers of the conference would later describe their reasoning behind the invitation list, which can be read as arguments for jurisdiction for various professions. Among the many threats to the "Sanctity of Life" in contemporary society, the organizers recognized a number "in the scientific area [which] were easily identified: contraception, abortion, eugenics, euthanasia, drug testing, and human experimentation." In light of this, "the biologists and medical scientists were absolutely essential [to invite.]" This sounds like scientists should have jurisdiction.

"But the scientists could not be allowed to have the picnic all to themselves; they should be exposed to counterpoint from enlightened non-scientists," continued the organizers. Contrary to the views of some scientists, the organizers felt that "values lie beyond the domain of science," seemingly a good sign for the theologians and a swipe at the jurisdictional aspirations of the scientists. Who, however, would be called upon to enlighten us about values? "Certainly law would be one discipline indispensable to the conference . . . [and] in light of contemporary moral concerns, an observer of man's social institutions and behavior—a sociologist—should be invited to comment on the relevance of this to the sanctity of life. Likewise, religion and philosophy could scarcely be overlooked."

This last sentence may imply a field of equal competitors, but the next sentence belies this. "There is such uncertainty about the force of religious belief in face of modern scientific inquiry that one might reasonably ask what the role of religious principles will be in guiding human behavior." That comment is not followed up, but is just allowed to dangle like an accusation. One gets the sense that the theologian was invited out of inertia, and that the organizers had wished to find a more plausible alternative. In a portentous comment for the future of these debates, the organizers declared that "since the entire discourse [of the conference] was well within the domain of philosophy," a philosopher was invited to comment at the end of the conference "in the hope that a final common path might be found, of reason, of arbitration (if necessary), and at least of common sense, if not pure logic." Perhaps theologians like Ramsey should have seen the writing on the wall, even at this early point.

That sociologist, Edward Shils, began the conference by summarizing the social conditions under which the question of the "sanctity of life" is to be examined. We must ask about the "sanctity of life," he wrote, because of "the decline of Christian belief about the place of man in the divine scheme and the consequent diminution of its force as a criterion in the judgement of the work and permissibility of human actions" (Shils 1968:2). Undeterred, the theologian at the conference, Ramsey, would make an argument for the immorality of abortion by translating theological claims, using references to scripture and Protestant theologian Karl Barth (Ramsey 1968). Clearly, the organizers of this conference thought other professions, like philosophy, were more deserving of jurisdiction.

A 1971 conference sent a similar discouraging message to theologians. One of the great opponents of the theologians was one of the inventors of in vitro fertilization, Robert Edwards. He was a forceful advocate of the idea of "scientific freedom," by which scientists could conduct their research without the interference of the public. ("Scientific freedom," using my terminology, simply means exclusive jurisdiction by scientists over the ethics of their actions.) In a later memoir, Edwards gives an account of his first encounter with Ramsey at a conference on in vitro fertilization in 1971. He wrote of Ramsey: "He had to be seen and heard to be believed. I had to endure a denunciation of our work as if from some nineteenth-century pulpit. . . . He had uttered sentiments in his rhetorical way that would not have disgraced those directed against Charles Darwin one hundred years earlier."

What is telling is not that Ramsey would have given a theologically based denunciation of Edwards' work, but Edwards' rendition of the response of the audience, which comprised "senators, judges, doctors, scientists and writers" (Edwards and Steptoe 1980:112). That is, these were a mix of the jurisdiction-givers (the elite public), who give or withhold jurisdiction through their response. People they do not approve of will not be given a soapbox again. Edwards wrote that "I had hardly begun my second sentence" of response to Ramsey: "— 'Dogma that has entered biology either from Communist or from Christian sources has done nothing but harm . . .'—when I was interrupted by huge applause. The audience were on their feet clapping. . . . [Ramsey's] point of view had been shatteringly rejected by the audience. Indeed he made no further contribution to that symposium" (Edwards and Steptoe 1980:114). In sum, it appeared that the audience, composed of those who could give jurisdiction over promulgating the ethics of science and medicine, was hostile to secular translations of explicitly theological ends, suggesting that a change in strategy would be necessary.

Faced with utter marginalization in the debate that they truly wanted to influence to further their theologically motivated ends, theologians took the risk of no longer discussing the theological ends they had translated and only using secular ends so that they could continue in the debate. According to Albert Jonsen, who was a Catholic priest during his early involvement in these debates, "early religious bioethicists . . . dispensed with their outward religious appearance in order to make themselves welcome and comprehensible to the secular world" (Jonsen 2006:34). There were several features of the social environment at the time that also encouraged this evolution.

Characteristics of the Jurisdiction-Givers

This was a debate in cultural bioethics, where the jurisdiction-givers were the gatekeepers to media, like newspaper reporters, book editors, and TV producers. Who was this "elite public"?

The United States has been religiously pluralistic from its founding. What matters to the case at hand is that pluralism among the general citizens did not come to be represented among societal elites until midway through the twentieth century, with the mainline Protestants having disproportionate influence. But, by the late 1960s it was clear that one could not assume that a generic mainline Protestant ethic was held by these elites.

Up until the 1950s, there were still "Jewish quotas" at Ivy League schools, genteel discrimination against non-Protestant faculty, and Catholic and Jewish hospitals existed as separate institutions with Catholic and Jewish doctors. By the 1960s people of non-Protestant backgrounds were not unusual in the professions due to a decline in outright discrimination and expansions in the availability of higher education. Simultaneously, in the 1960s, college enrollments were surging as government funding increased, making college and professional educations no longer primarily the province of mainline Protestants (Wuthnow 1988:86).

Scholars have examined various indicators of the disproportionate influence of one religious group over another, such as looking at the religious affiliation of those listed in *Who's Who*, professional societies, members of Congress, or government elites (Davidson, Pyle and Reyes 1995; Davidson 1994), or looking at just who is getting college degrees (Wuthnow 1988). The story is the same from the mid-century forward: the elites in society increasingly "look like the society," religiously speaking. Whereas half a century ago most elites were Episcopalians, Congregationalists, Presbyterians, and Unitarians (i.e., mainline Protestants), now many are Jews, Catholics, and evangelicals such as Southern Baptists, Adventists, Nazarenes, and Pentecostals.

Ramsey, for example, came to experience this pluralism first-hand as he moved into debates on science and medicine. In 1969 he was invited to give a prestigious series of lectures at Yale Divinity School, which were later published as his most influential work, *The Patient as Person*. He notes the long string of Protestant theologians who had been invited over the centuries to give these lectures—among the most recognizable are Henry Sloan Coffin, Harry Emerson Fosdick, and Reinhold Niebuhr—and notes that his lectures would be unique in the history of the series. They would be co-sponsored by the medical school, and "on each of the four nights, I would be joined by a panel of commentators, consisting of physicians and medical school professors and theologians—Protestant, Catholic and Jewish." He would not only be confronted with this theological pluralism, but he also decided that he would do the theological equivalent of fieldwork. "I judged at once, or course, that I needed to know how medical men themselves discuss the questions they confront," and arranged to be tutored at (Catholic) Georgetown University Hospital during the spring semesters in 1968 and 1969 on how doctors made decisions.

His invitation to observe physicians at work came from André Hellegers, an active Catholic obstetrician-gynecologist (Ramsey 1970b:xx). In the book that resulted from the lectures, he most effusively thanked Hellegers and a Jewish physician, biologist, and philosopher named Leon Kass for their reading of the chapters. In an earlier time, Kass would not have been in his prestigious post at the National Academy of Sciences to encounter Ramsey, and Hellegers would not have expected a Protestant to be interested in the workings of a Catholic hospital. Yet, times had changed. Ramsey would state in the preface to *The Patient as Person* that "an increasing number of moralists—Catholic, Protestant, Jewish and unlabeled men—are manifesting interest, devoting their trained powers of ethical reasoning to questions of medical practice and technology" (Ramsey 1970b:xvi). Given the religious diversity, explicit translations of particular and explicit theological ends was looking less and less plausible as a strategy for getting past the gatekeepers of the public sphere, and influencing what actually occurs in science and medicine.

This tension was evident in *The Patient as Person* itself. While above I described the translation this book engaged in, other analysts have concluded that the book was not really too explicit about the theological ends that were being translated. Theologian Stanley Hauerwas claims he used to kid Ramsey—with a form of kidding that was clearly a critique—that "all the theology in *The Patient as Person* was in the preface" (Hauerwas 1996:66).

Characteristics of the Theologians

It was not simply the growing perception of pluralism among the jurisdiction-givers that resulted in the theologians' retreating from the explicit discussion of explicitly theological ends. There were forces in the theological profession itself that led to weakness. Most notably, to necessarily oversimplify, theology was divided along a continuum from those on one end, who translated explicitly theological ends, to those on the other, who were committed to an almost entirely secular form of theology. This latter end of the spectrum will probably sound strange to people unfamiliar with this era. However, in the 1960s there were movements in both liberal Protestantism and Catholicism toward a form of theology that was accessible to all people, whether or not they believed in God.

Among Protestants, from the situation-ethics wing came what has become known as "death of God" theology. In Harvey Cox's influential version of this thesis, God had freed humans through secularization, and they must now live with the implications of this freedom

(Laney 1970:18). The "death of God" advocates and the "situationists" would both "eliminate any exclusively Christian conditions or terms" from what was also called "the new morality" (Laney 1970:19). To slightly overstate the case, the claim was that there was nothing unique about Christian ethics that could not be obtained through secular sources.

Among Catholics, a similar strand of thinking had emerged. Reacting to neo-scholasticism, by the early 1970s a variant of natural law theology had emerged that Vincent MacNamara calls "an autonomous ethic" theology.[6] It goes beyond the purposes of this chapter to delve into the history of Catholic theology, but a quote from one of the advocates sums up the view of this new school well: "Christian morality . . . is basically and substantially a human morality, that is a morality of true manhood. That means that truth, honesty and fidelity, in their materiality, are not specifically Christian but universally human values. . . ."[7] As one critic at the time stated, "whereas a few years previously theologians regarded it as natural to demand that the teaching of morality should be theological, i.e., 'Conceived in terms of scripture and of salvation history' things have been entirely reversed 'so that Christian morality is understood in rational, philosophical terms, i.e., in terms of empirical human science.'"[8] There was then no reason to describe any theological ends, or even to translate at all.

Even in the first period, the Catholic contributions to bioethical debate were approximately halfway between the types of arguments made in the second and third eras. In theologian James Gustafson's words, in Catholic natural law theology, "ethical analysis and prescription was theological in principle; moralists were theologians by being moralists. Enough said about theology" (Gustafson 1978:387).

In addition to the conflict in theology between theologians who translated to secular ends and those who started and ended with secular claims, there was conflict about the religious nature of "scientific progress" itself. For example, a number of theologians at the time were perceived, at least by the Ramsey wing of the theological profession, as total apologists for a scientific and not a theological worldview. The divisions within the theological house were well described by Ramsey, who complained of Catholic theologian Karl Rahner, "Roman Catholic omega-pointers" (a reference to the omega-point theory of French Jesuit de Chardin), and "Protestant theologians of secular, historical 'hope' who collapse the distinction between being men before God and being God before we have learned to be men" (Ramsey 1970a:142). The gist of this new theology was that humans, created by God, had used their God-given powers to engage in Godlike activity, such as creating new life forms. An ally of Ramsey, Leon Kass, would call these theologians "theologians-turned-technocrats" who "sanctify the new freedoms: 'what can be done, should be done'" (Kass 1972:60).

Ramsey would have similar things to say about the situation ethics being promoted at the time by theologians such as Joseph Fletcher. Fletcher, who was personally beginning to secularize by this point (Fletcher 1993), would say that "if the greatest good of the greatest number . . . were served by it, it would be justifiable not only to specialize the capacities of people by cloning or by constructive genetic engineering, but also to bio-engineer or bio-design parahumans or 'modified men'" (Fletcher 1971:779). As Ramsey would quip, this type of reasoning "sounds remarkably like a priestly blessing over everything, doing duty for ethics" (Ramsey 1970a:139–140). The implication for the theologians' attempt at jurisdiction is that it is hard to win the jurisdictional battle with science when some of your soldiers are using the language of your enemy, seemingly blessing scientific activity as an end in itself.

A second internal problem for the theologians was a lack of resources. The best resource for the theologians would have been access to the members of their respective traditions, because they could have influenced gatekeepers through their purchases of books, subscriptions to magazines, and so on. But, because these first critics of the scientists were by and large not employed by denominations themselves but rather were academic theologians, public intellectuals, or lay activists, this direct access was not open to them. Among the Protestants, none of these issues was discussed in the denominations, with the exception of a limited discussion about abortion. These Protestants were not theologians who wrote Sunday school materials, but people who wrote scholarly journal articles.

The explanation of why the Catholic theologians did not have access to the denominational machinery and ordinary Catholics is a bit more complex. To begin with, it is important to know that many of the earliest theologically oriented critics of the scientists were also involved with liberal politics within the Catholic Church. The second Vatican Council was occurring between 1962 and 1965, and in 1963 a small group was appointed by Pope John XXIII to review the Catholic position on contraception. One member of that group was Catholic layperson and obstetrician-gynecologist André Hellegers (who would later invite Ramsey to study at Georgetown).

Watching the birth control debate was a Catholic public intellectual with a Ph.D. in philosophy named Daniel Callahan, who was editor of the Catholic intellectual journal *Commonweal*. He, like Hellegers, was a liberal on the contraception debate, calling contraception "a test case for the contemporary renewal of the Church" (Walters 1985:9). In 1968, Pope Paul VI, through the release of *Humanae Vitae*, rejected the recommendations of the Papal Commission and reiterated the traditional stance of the Roman Catholic Church against contraception.

Hellegers was "deeply disappointed by the Pope's decision" (Walters 1985:9). Callahan was "equally distressed by *Humanae Vitae*," and the next year he edited a book called *The Catholic Case for Contraception* for the "express purpose of supporting the moral arguments of couples who dissented from *Humane Vitae*" (Walters 1985:10). He would also cofound the first institutional home for the growing movement challenging science and medicine—the Institute of Society, Ethics, and the Life Sciences (later renamed the Hastings Center).

In 1971, Hellegers founded the Joseph and Rose Kennedy Institute for the Study of Human Reproduction and Bioethics at Georgetown

University and recruited an ecumenical group of Christian scholars to staff it. LeRoy Walters, interpreting these events, traces Hellegers's "determination to find a non-ecclesiastical forum for the ongoing exploration of problems at the interface of biology, medicine and moral theology" to his reaction to *Humanae Vitae* (Walters 1985:10). Three Catholic priests deeply involved in the earliest moments of bioethical debate—Albert Jonsen, Charles McCarthy, and Warren Reich—all left the priesthood at least partly because they could not "continue to accept and be obedient to the moral authority of the Church" due to *Humanae Vitae* (Fox and Swazey 2008:65). Thus, in the Catholic component of the theological challenge, the institutions that began to solidify the movement after the "decade of conferences" were already committed to a separation of their work from the institutional church, due to their being on the losing side of *Humanae Vitae* and other issues. The resources of the institutional church and direct access to the laity would not be available to them.

The Result: A Debate About (Secularly Expressed) Ends

Theology was weak. Its particularism was out of touch with the growing pluralism of the elite public who would provide jurisdiction. Theologians were also divided among themselves, and disconnected from their traditional bases of resources. No one group of theologians, speaking theologically, was up to the jurisdictional challenge from the scientists. The threats to humanity at the time seemed strong enough to justify some compromises in one's theological language in order to win the war.

The compromise in Period 2 was that theologians would debate secular ends that were presumably condensed translations of their theological ends, but the theological part went unmentioned. This made the arguments more suitable for widespread communication. It is important to note that starting with theology and translating to secular ends resulted in a large number of diverse ends' being expressed in the overall debate.

By 1978, theologian James Gustafson described the abandonment of the explicit, condensed translations of theological ends championed by Ramsey and the rise of theologians talking only about secular ends with the connection to theological ends at best implicit. He wrote that it is clear that people with theological *training* were writing in public bioethical debate:

> whether *theology* is thereby in interaction with these areas, however, is less clear. For some writers the theological authorization for the ethical principles and procedures they use is explicit; this is clearly the case for the most prolific and polemical of the Protestants, Paul Ramsey. For others, writing as "ethicists," the relation of their moral discourse to any specific theological principles, or even to a definable religious outlook is opaque. Indeed, in response to a query from a friend (who is a distinguished philosopher) about how the term "ethicist" has come about, I responded in a pejorative way, "An ethicist is a former theologian who does not have the professional credentials of a moral philosopher."
>
> Much of the writing in the field is by persons who desire to be known as "religious ethicists" if only to distinguish themselves for practical reasons from those holding cards in the philosophers' union. Exactly what the adjective "religious" refers to, however, is far from obvious. . . . Again Ramsey is to be commended; one can ask for nothing more forthright than his 1974 declaration, "I always write as the ethicist I am, namely a Christian ethicist, and not as some hypothetical common denominator" (Gustafson 1978:386).

Gustafson sees (again in my terminology) that the problem is that the professionals who are the jurisdiction-providers do not care about theology: "Most of the professional persons the writers seek to influence are judged not to be interested in the theological grounds from which the moral and analysis and prescription grows" (Gustafson 1978:387).

While not obviously religious, religious ends were still driving the conclusions if these were actually implicit condensed translations. For example, Joseph Fletcher would move from a utilitarian maximization of the theological concept of *agape* in the 1960s to a utilitarian maximization of the secular-sounding end of *happiness* in the 1970s. Fletcher's 1966 *Situation Ethics* is essentially an argument that decisions in medicine and science should follow a "consequentialist" maximization of *agape*. There he states that the two principles to be maximized are from the apostle Paul: " 'The written code kills, but the Spirit gives life' (II Cor. 3:6), and 'For the whole law is fulfilled in one word, 'You shall love your neighbor as yourself' (Gal. 5:14)" (Fletcher 1966:30). By the 1970s, maximizing "love your neighbor as yourself" (*agape*) had become maximizing utility.

Similarly, consider Kass' remark about human cloning: "For man is the watershed which divides the world into those things that belong to nature and those that are made by men. To lay one's hands on human generation is to take a major step toward making man himself simply another of the man-made things" (Kass 1972:54). Kass's end could be called "no instrumental modification of humans." Here is a conundrum that scientists do not usually like to think about, but it was *the* topic of conversation among theologians and their fellow travelers, yet all without reference to explicit theology.[9] For example, Callahan would respond to Kass by asking "whether man's humanity can survive" new technologies such as in vitro fertilization. He noted that scientists probably "believe that their work is both praiseworthy and intensively human. To seek knowledge is human. To improve man's lot is human. To make things, even human beings, is human." He called for further debate over "some general, comprehensive, and universal norms for 'the human'" (Callahan 1972:97–99). Theologians were still trying to keep this discussion in their jurisdiction with this secular debate about the ends we should be pursuing through technology.

So, during this second era, theologians would debate the ends we should pursue and whether the proposed technologies are consistent with these ends. They would think through the question in their "first voice" of theology and explicitly argue for a secular end, with the theological part remaining in the background. However, even this method of using condensed translations of theological ends was not to last long.

Gustafson was standing between the peaks of the second and third eras—he was writing out of concern for the lost theological voice of the first era, but was witnessing the advent of the third. Many of the religious ethicists were beginning to ask thin little questions about problems that had been defined by scientists and physicians that did not require a discussion of ends at all but assumed an end. An example was: "Should one cut the power source to a respirator for Patient Y whose circumstances are a, b and c? [which] is not utterly dissimilar to asking whether $8.20 an hour or $8.55 an hour ought to be paid to carpenter's helpers in Kansas City" (Gustafson 1978:387). The explicitly theological defense of their jurisdiction had lasted only a few years, until they began the second era of debating secular ends that were implicit condensed translations of theological ends. This seemed like an effective strategy for maintaining jurisdiction for the theologians. They were speaking a secular language, attempting to be understood by all participants in the public sphere. However, this strategy would only last a few years more as a shift in the jurisdiction-providers made the theologians' secular condensed translation methods obsolete.

Notes

1. Certainly at least Christian theologians have a long history of translating theological ideas into a secular idiom for communication with those outside of the tradition. Indeed, Christian biblical scholarship concludes that each of the Synoptic Gospels (Matthew, Mark, and Luke)

were, in my terms, condensed translations of the Jesus story meant to appeal to different audiences, such as Jews or Gentiles.

2. While there is consensus about the centrality of religious elites in the formation of bioethical debate, the primary scholarly debate is whether these religiously identified elites ever spoke theologically, or whether they simply were theologians making secular philosophical arguments (Jonsen 2006:33; Messikomer, Fox and Swazey 2001; Childress 2003). I will argue below that there was indeed an explicitly religious era.

3. I would say that Paul Ramsey would be the possible exception to this generalization. Others, such as Hauerwas, see him as the quintessential Niebuhrian liberal (Hauerwas 1996).

4. Before turning to medical issues, Ramsey was well known for basic theology and just war theory. There are many summaries of Ramsey's work. See Long 1993; Attwood 1992; Smith 1993; Tubbs 1996; and Hauerwas 1997:Ch. 8.

5. Ramsey, according to one of his critics, held "the conviction that Christianity had formed something called Western civilization, which continued to bear the marks of the Gospel" (Hauerwas 1997:128).

6. Neo-scholasticism in Catholic ethics produced a stream of moral manuals that have, according to one account, "a great air of security and certainty," reflecting "a confident understanding of the identity of Christian morality." Oversimplifying, the whole point of them is to make sure you get to heaven (MacNamara 1985:9, 10).

7. Josef Fuchs, writing in 1970, quoted in MacNamara (1985:40).

8. Gustav Ermecke, writing in 1972, quoted in MacNamara (1985:55).

9. Kass was not a theologian, but was in the same debating community as the theologians (Evans 2002:Ch. 2).

Chapter 2

The Theological Retreat
and the Emergence of the
Bioethics Profession

The struggle between the scientists and the theologians in the 1960s and early 1970s set the groundwork for much more momentous changes in the 1970s. Changes in the jurisdiction-providers destabilized the competition, and allowed the new profession of bioethics to emerge and quickly take jurisdiction over three task-spaces, as the theologians and scientists retreated. The theologians and their allies were essentially victims of their own success. They had loudly questioned where scientists were going with technologies like organ transplantation, and the public finally began to pay attention. In fact, they were paying so much attention that these issues soon caught the eye of elected officials, who began to suggest various legislative remedies to force scientists and physicians to adhere to the basic ethical insights that were being generated by the early bioethical debate.

The government established itself as the jurisdiction-giver over a new task, public policy bioethics. More or less simultaneously, the government also inserted itself as the jurisdiction-provider for the research bioethics, and a few years later the government became the jurisdiction-provider for health-care ethics consultation. Both the research bioethics and health-care ethics consultation task-spaces had long been under the jurisdiction of science/medicine.

The Research Bioethics Task Space

Most of the debate I described in the previous chapter was about revolutionary new technologies like in vitro fertilization, cloning, and mind control, but a somewhat separate controversy had started earlier with the more long-standing issue of human experimentation. In the 1950s, scientists had strong jurisdiction over research bioethics. In fact, it was so strong that it was not considered a separate task of scientists. Historian David Rothman concludes that "American researchers in the immediate post–World War II period ran their laboratories free of external constraints. The autonomy they enjoyed in conducting human experiments was limited only by their individual consciences" (Rothman 1991:69). However, they soon began to feel a threat to their exclusive jurisdiction.

In the 1950s, the US government set up a hospital to conduct medical research on healthy human subjects at the National Institutes of Health (NIH) in Bethesda, Maryland. The researchers were very worried about public appearances and pressure from elected officials, and worried that some scandal would cut off their funding stream. Government lawyers suggested that they would be less liable if they made sure they had the written consent of their experimental subjects. But the scientists wanted to minimize the situations in which they had to obtain the written consent of the research subjects to be experimented upon, and wanted to instead rely on the good character of the researcher to ensure that research subjects would be treated well. It was typical during this time to argue that research subjects had given implicit consent by coming to the hospital, or that they could give oral consent to someone on the research team. In other words, research bioethics was ideally not even a separate task, but just part of being a good scientist or doctor. There were minimal ethical guidelines in place—it was just presumed that a group of research physicians would practice good judgement. However, to stave off outside pressure, the NIH set up a committee of fellow researchers to make sure that the research protocol would not violate the rights of research subjects (this was essentially the first institutional review board [IRB]).

This was a process only for the Clinical Center at the NIH in Bethesda. However, alongside the debates described in the last chapter, public scandals in human-subjects research had been emerging throughout the 1960s—not at the NIH in Bethesda, but at other institutions whose research was funded by the NIH. For example, journalists broke the story in 1964 that NIH-funded researchers at New York's Jewish Chronic Disease Hospital had injected 22 patients with cancer cells without first getting their consent (Stark 2012: 145). An implication of the media articles on these scandals was that the public should wonder whether—to use my terminology—research scientists should have jurisdiction over the ethics of their experiments.

Lawyers at the NIH amplified a long-standing concern that the NIH could be legally responsible for the unethical behavior of NIH grantees, and a senator from New York, Jacob Javits, was pressing the NIH to address this issue. Their solution to this legal liability by 1966 was to essentially export the NIH Clinical Center IRB model, requiring any institution that received NIH funding to set up such a committee (Advisory Committee on Human Radiation Experiments 1996:100). A committee at each institution would be morally and legally responsible for research, and could determine its own ethical standards and procedures for enacting the widely accepted practice of obtaining some form of consent (Stark 2012: 154). This policy was later given regulatory status in 1974 after being promulgated by the Department of Health, Education and Welfare.

Through this process, the scientists and physicians had done a fairly good job of maintaining jurisdiction in the face of public pressure. Scientists and physicians still controlled the local committees, and it was their ethics that would still be paramount. As a memo from the Surgeon General to grantees said in 1966: "the wisdom and sound professional judgment of you and your staff will determine what constitutes the rights and welfare of human subjects in research, what constitutes informed consent, and what constitutes the risks and potential medical benefits of a particular investigation."[1] A separate research bioethics task-space had been created, but the scientists had jurisdiction, and the profession itself could remove its bad apples.[2] However, the creation of a distinct task-space made jurisdiction over this task open to challenge.

The Health-Care Ethics Consultation Task-Space

As of the 1950s and early 1960s, medicine had rock-solid jurisdiction over the ethics of the administration of health care in medical settings. Indeed, this jurisdiction had been solidifying for hundreds of years. As historian David Rothman states, "from the classical age onward, the most distinguishing characteristic of medical ethics was the extent to which it was monopolized by practicing physicians, not by formal philosophers" (Rothman 1991:102). However, he continues, there was a revolution in the public's view of bedside ethics between 1966 and 1976, wherein "the new rules for the laboratory," by which he means the ethical system used in the research bioethics jurisdiction, "permeated the examining room, circumscribing the discretionary authority of the individual physician" (Rothman 1991:107).

In the 1960s there were glimmers of outsiders' being let into the ethical decision-making in hospital environments. In Seattle in 1962, a committee of the general public was formed to make decisions about which patients would be given access to a new kidney-dialysis technique in short supply. If patients did not receive treatment, they would die (Rothman 1991:150). Also, individual humanists were allowed into medical education in the 1960s and 1970s, and were brought in on an ad hoc basis to give advice on ethics (Bosk 2008:43; Fletcher, Quist and Jonsen 1989:12). However, doctors generally resisted trespassers on their jurisdiction.

As in human experimentation, a series of public scandals perhaps made the loss of jurisdiction by physicians inevitable as they were increasingly seen as not being able to keep their own ethical house in order. In 1973 there was a public report critical of the treatment of patients in the neonatal intensive care unit at Yale-New Haven Hospital (Bosk 2008:42). Some reformers in the cultural bioethical debate described in the last chapter began to call for ethics committees to help physicians with their decisions. One of the proposals came from Karen Teel, who, writing in 1975, called for hospital ethics committees comprising "physicians, social workers, attorneys and theologians" (Teel 1975:9). That theologians were mentioned (and not philosophers)—and that she noted that such existing committees were irreverently called "God squads"—suggests that the theologians were pushing back against science and medicine in this jurisdiction as well.

The Emergence of the Public Policy Bioethics Task-Space

As early as 1968, Senator Walter Mondale had held hearings on setting up a government commission to oversee research in areas such as genetic engineering, organ transplantation, behavior control, experimentation on humans, and the financing of research. Like the theologians, Mondale was interested in the deep questions. He started the hearings by saying: "Recent medical advances raise grave and fundamental ethical and legal questions for our society. Who shall live and who shall die? How long shall life be preserved and how should it be altered? Who will make decisions? How shall society be prepared?" (Jonsen 1998:90–91).

Scientists were fearful that the cascade of research money that had come their way since the 1950s would either slow to a trickle as the public became fearful of the fruit of scientific investigations, or that the money would come with strings attached, like the Congress determining what experiments could and could not be done. They blamed this new attention not only on their scientific colleagues who had been trying to expand their jurisdiction into the task-space traditionally held by theology, who were advocating utopian scientific visions of refiguring the meaning of life, which had scared the public, but also on the theologians and others whom these visions had lured into the debate. Writing specifically about human genetic engineering, Harvard bacteriologist Bernard Davis wrote in 1970 that the "exaggeration of the dangers from genetics will inevitably contribute to an already distorted public view, which increasingly blames science for our problems and ignores its contributions to our welfare." This "irresponsible hyperbole" of the previous generation of scientists "has already influenced the funding of research. . . . If, in panic, our society should curtail fundamental genetic research, we would pay a huge price" (Davis 1970:1279, 1282). He finished with a call to arms for the scientists against theologians and other challengers, writing that "genetics will surely survive the current attacks, just as it survived attacks from the Communist Party in Moscow and from fundamentalists in Tennessee. But meanwhile . . . we may have to defend vigorously the value of objective and verifiable knowledge, especially when it comes into conflict with political, theological or sociological dogmas" (Davis 1970:1283).

Scientists began a retreat, abandoning attempts to establish the purpose of medical and scientific technologies to the theologians. However, they retreated carefully in order to minimize the damage to their other jurisdictions. Scientists involved in the debates about broader and more innovative technologies like human genetic engineering saw committees like they had established in research bioethics as a way of seeming to address the public's concerns while limiting the actual influence others would have on their work. They suggested setting up various government advisory committees where the citizens could fulminate about their concerns, but would be unable to actually constrain scientists. Edwards, the in vitro fertilization pioneer introduced above, would say that biologists must "invent a method of taking counsel of mankind" or "society will thrust its advice on biologists . . . in a manner or form seriously hampering to science." What was needed was an organization "easily approached and consulted to advise and assist biologists and others to reach *their own* decisions."[3]

This attempt to limit others' influence would not hold, and the scientists' and physicians' jurisdictions would not last. Continued revelations made it perhaps inevitable that the state would establish itself as the jurisdiction-giver and eventually select a profession other than science/medicine for the three jurisdictions. In the research bioethics task-space, in 1972, years after the formation of the proto-IRBs controlled by scientists, it was revealed that the U.S. Public Health Service had been conducting a 40-year-long experiment where a group of about 600 poor and uneducated black men in Tuskegee, Alabama, with syphilis were left untreated. The idea was to autopsy them when they died to see the effect of syphilis on the human body. When combined with other revelations that physicians in hospitals had been experimenting on ordinary patients without their knowledge, Congress felt compelled to do something. Historian David Rothman concludes that it was public attention to scandals in human experimentation, such as the Tuskegee experiment, that provided the final impetus for government intervention into the ethics of researchers (Rothman 1991:182–89)

Congress could have, as the scientists feared, directly looked to what *they* perceived as the values of the nation and banned certain technologies and certain practices. They could have become, themselves, the regulator of science and medicine. But they did not. They first created the task of public policy bioethics, and established the government as the jurisdiction-giver, by creating the first commission whose task was to suggest ethical policy to the government. At the same time as they created the commission, they legally established that the research bioethics task would be under the control of federal policy.

This transformation began in 1973 when Senator Edward Kennedy held hearings on bills to regulate human experimentation and introduced a bill to create a National Human Experimentation Board. The scientists were still fighting for local control, opposing what we would now call a national-level IRB, trying to defend their jurisdiction over research bioethics. When it became clear that the scientists would be successful in blocking Kennedy's bill, Kennedy introduced the bill that would become the National Research Act. The Act created the National Commission for the Protection of Human Subjects of Biomedical and Behavioral Research in return for the Department of Health Education and Welfare's issuing human-subject research regulations (Advisory Committee on Human Radiation Experiments 1996:103). According to one history of this era, "The trade-off was clear: no national regulatory body in return for regulations applying to the research funded or performed by the government agency responsible for the greatest proportion of human subject research" (Advisory Committee on Human Radiation Experiments 1996:103). Such regulations were issued in 1974 mandating the creation of an IRB at institutions receiving money from the Department of Health, Education and Welfare.

Perhaps more important for my narrative, the law created the National Commission, which first met in 1974. In my terms, this was the first institution in public policy bioethics. One of the mandated tasks of the Commission was to "conduct a comprehensive investigation and study to identify the basic ethical principles which should underlie the conduct of biomedical and behavioral research involving human subjects" and "develop guidelines which should be followed in such research to assure that it is conducted in accord with such principles."[4] In other words, they were to create the ethical system for research bioethics that could be put into public law, to replace the ethics used by the scientists whom the public seemingly no longer trusted. That the government had forced researchers to use IRBs, and called for the creation of this ethical system, indicates it was now the jurisdiction-giver over research bioethics.

The National Commission contained a few theologians among the physicians, social scientists, and others. They created a number of reports, and towards the end of the Commission's life, they worked on articulating those general ethical principles for use in research bioethics. By their own description, they decided in a series of meetings, through scholarly reflection, that there were three primary principles "among those generally accepted in our cultural tradition" that were at stake in human experimentation: respect for persons, beneficence, and justice. These three principles justified the practices of informed consent, risk-benefit analysis, and the selection of research subjects, respectively, and were published in 1979 as The Belmont Report (National Commission for the Protection of Human Subjects of Biomedical and Behavioral Research 1978a). These principles were later given the force of law for research conducted with federal money.

Selecting these principles revealed that the scientists' retreat continued to be fairly damage-free. These principles were actually not a profound challenge to the scientists' jurisdiction in research bioethics, as the elaboration of these principles was a post hoc philosophical backfilling of justifications for practices scientists had supposedly endorsed for many years (Faden and Beauchamp 1986: 216). For example, in 1966, the Department of Health, Education and Welfare regulations required of grantee institutions that they address three topics in their evaluation of research: "an independent determination (1) of the rights and welfare of the individual or individual involved, (2) of the appropriateness of the methods used to secure informed consent, and (3) of the risks and potential medical benefits of the investigation" (Advisory Committee on Human Radiation Experiments 1996:100). This was essentially mandating informed consent, now justified by the principle of respect for persons, and risk-benefit analysis, now justified by the principle of beneficence. Of course, the background justifications for the practices *did* change. For example, whereas it is clear that one "principle" behind the scientists' practice of written informed consent for patients who were also subject to research in the 1950s and 1960s was to avoid being sued (Advisory Committee on Human Radiation Experiments 1996; Stark 2012: Chapter 6), now informed consent was justified in reference to the more philosophical principle of respect for persons. But changing the philosophical justification for the practice would not directly change what scientists ideally did.

This commission essentially created the system of abstract knowledge the bioethics profession uses in all of its jurisdictions, and thus is the origin of the profession itself. In the Belmont Report, this body had not decided what the ethics of the public *should be* regarding a public issue, and did not follow the ethics of some subgroup in the population, but instead claimed to have channeled *existing* values of all citizens in such a way that the values of the public could be used to create public policy—in this case, human-research-subjects policy of the executive branch. The scientists' ethics had been portrayed as being in opposition to the public's ethics, but bioethicists, representing the public, would soon take jurisdiction from the scientists and physicians in three of the four task-spaces.

Government Jurisdiction Over Health-Care Ethics Consultation

As the primary user of its product, the government was now the jurisdiction-provider for public policy bioethics. It was also, by legislative mandate, the jurisdiction-provider for research bioethics, and professions would have to adhere to the government's interests and predilections to obtain jurisdiction. A few years later, and much more slowly and episodically, the government became a jurisdiction-provider in health-care ethics consultation. While they resisted intrusion longer, the physicians' jurisdiction was severely damaged by the 1976 legal decision about Karen Quinlan, when the court was asked to decide whether her life-support should be ended (Veatch 1977; Bosk 2010:S138; Fletcher, Quist and Jonsen 1989). Citing the proposal of Teel, the court "suggested that hospitals form ethics committees to keep disputes, such as the one before them, out of the courts" (Bosk 2008:42). That only started progress toward creating a system to bring non-doctors "to the bedside" to give ethical advice, but the next burst of activity was another scandal in the early 1980s surrounding the cases of a number of severely disabled newborns who were supposedly left to die (Bosk 2008:43). "Infant Doe" regulations were promulgated by the Department of Health and Human Services, and following the recommendations of the American Academy of Pediatrics and others, the regulations strongly encouraged, but did not mandate, that hospitals establish infant-care review committees (Cranford and Doudera 1984:13).

In 1983 a government ethics commission (to be discussed below) produced a report calling for the ethical review of medical decisions via mechanisms "such as 'ethics committees'" (Cranford and Doudera 1984:13). Despite these calls, as they were not yet mandated by the state, there were few ethics committees in place. A study in the early 1980s estimated that just one percent of the country's hospitals had ethics committees (although there were a few more at Catholic hospitals) (Cranford and Doudera 1984:14–15). However, the presence of health-care ethics consultation, particularly in the form of committees, has grown during the subsequent decades, now that a direct government mandate is in place, with the Joint Commission on the Accreditation of Health Care Organizations requiring that hospitals have some ethics mechanism (Bosk 2010:S138). By 2000, nearly all hospitals with more than 100 beds provided health-care ethics consultation (Fox, Myers and Pearlman 2007:15). That said, the government has used a lighter hand in its jurisdiction-giving than in research bioethics, and hospital administrators also provide jurisdiction for the time being by deciding how to design their ethics consultation services.

Methods in the Bioethics Profession's System of Abstract Knowledge

These newly configured task-spaces with the new jurisdiction-provider shook up the professional competition for jurisdiction. Alongside the profession of theology, the profession of philosophy had increasingly come to be represented in these debates, viewing bioethics as a type of applied ethics. Philosophical thought influenced the first commission, and a new profession of bioethics emerged from this commission with a new system of abstract knowledge that was influenced by, yet distinct from, a particular type of philosophy. This new system and the attendant methods of the bioethics profession were ideally suited for the new jurisdiction-provider.

The first commission implicitly relied on a method that continues to be used by government ethics commissions, often in conjunction with other methods called "consensus among diverse commissioners." The idea is that through the use of consensus in decision-making in a group of diverse commissioners, the group's decision will reflect the ethics of all Americans (Moreno 1995). Put simply, if a group cannot reach consensus, then they have not reached the common morality on the ethical problem, but rather diverse and potentially irreconcilable positions. In the words of the executive director of the President's Commission (1979–1983) consensus "encourages the commissioners to seek the common ground that best expresses the moral insights and values of Americans today, in light of our shared, albeit not uniform, religious and philosophical traditions" (Capron 1983:8).

Consensus is claimed to generate the common morality because the commissioners are diverse, coming from a range of professions and demographic groups. For example, the Office of Technology Assessment, discussing what makes a successful bioethics commission, states that "diversity in race, ethnicity, gender, and professional experience is a paramount factor in appointing commissioners and staff. Ethics involves values, and a commission with monolithic membership or staffing cannot hope to adequately represent the diverse range of perspectives in American society" (U.S. Congress 1993:34).

Common-Morality Principlism

To return to the history of professional competition, the consensus method developed by the first bioethicists was actually not too much of a problem for at least the theologians engaged in condensed translation, as they could be one of the diverse groups at the table debating their secular translations. After all, it is not unconstitutional for a theologian to advise a government agency, as long as the resulting policy itself does make the government appear to be endorsing a religious belief. However, critical for our understanding of why the bioethics profession gained its jurisdictions is the method of "common-morality principlism" that is either used on its own or in conjunction with consensus. Common-morality principlism has been by far the most influential method of the bioethicists, and unlike the others, is used in all of their jurisdictions. There are other methods that are used to articulate the common morality that do not rely on principles such as casuistry (Turner 2003:197), but there is no need here to describe every method used by bioethicists.[5]

The first bioethics commission identified three ethical principles that the public implicitly held concerning human experimentation. In and of itself, the development of three ends to maximize in human subjects research was not a challenge to the theologians if they had wanted to compete for jurisdiction over research bioethics. Participating theologians were already used to speaking a secular language, and these principles were probably good condensed translations of theological concerns, as exemplified by the discussion of Ramsey's view of respect for persons in previous pages. While each tradition could have came up with additional ends to consider for human experimentation, this was not a path that was inherently destructive to the theologians, and if this was to be the way public policy bioethics operated, theologians could have competed for jurisdiction.

The problem for the theological profession's competition with the nascent bioethics profession came from elsewhere. At the same time that the National Commission was trying to create its common-morality principles for the government to use for research bioethics, an employee of the Commission's—philosopher Tom L. Beauchamp—was co-authoring a textbook with a consultant to the

Commission—theologian James Childress—that would use the same principle-based approach for the ethics of *any* medical or scientific issue in the public policy bioethics jurisdiction, as well as for the research bioethics and nascent health-care ethics consultation jurisdictions (Beauchamp 2005). The principles in the textbook were the same as those the National Commission designed for use in research bioethics, except that the textbook split "beneficence" into "beneficence" and "non-maleficence," and "respect for persons" became the related "respect for autonomy," with the new list of commonly held principles being autonomy, beneficence, non-maleficence, and justice.[6]

I consider these articulated principles to be like the ends component of an ethical argument I described in the last chapter. These principles are a statement about what is of value, and research must be consistent with or maximize these values (depending on one's perspective). While principles have different meanings in philosophical and bioethical theory, in practical use by ordinary bioethics professionals, they take on this simplified meaning (Fox and Swazey 2008:169–70; Devettere 1995), becoming a list of societal ends that should be satisfied through medical research.[7] Therefore, and for example, research on human subjects is ethical if the research subjects' autonomy is respected (by obtaining their informed consent), beneficence is followed (by ensuring the experiment provides a positive risk:benefit ratio), and the research subjects are selected in a just manner (by, for example, not focusing on people who lack economic power).

Principlism fits as a method in the system of abstract knowledge of the bioethics profession because principlism assumes that the principles represent "the common morality."[8] According to Beauchamp and Childress, the "common morality" "comprises all and only those norms that all morally serious persons accept as authoritative" (2001:3). They also argue that it is "an institutional fact about morality, not merely our view of it, that it contains fundamental precepts" that function above the particularity of subcultures (2001:4).

Principlism was not invented to be a tool in jurisdictional competition, but was invented because the inventors believed it was the best way to make ethical decisions. This aspiration for a common-morality-based ethics was not only central to the philosophical tradition that Beauchamp was embedded in, but was an aspiration among the most liberal of theologians in this era, some of whom were involved in creating this nonreligious ethical system, and who would break off from theology to be among the first bioethicists. Creating a secular and universal ethical system not only fit with the Catholic natural law theory, and the "death of God theology" of some liberal Protestants at the time, but also the Quakerism of co-inventor James Childress (Evans 2002:85–89; Campbell 1993).

Common-morality principlism was extremely damaging to theologians because of *another* universal claim in principlism that draws more from philosophical than theological origins. The principles were argued to not only be universally held by all the citizens of the United States (or even the world), and to be *the* ends to pursue for human experimentation in research bioethics, but most critically they were also declared *the* universal ends applicable to all issues in science and medicine, such as health-care ethics consultation, cloning, human genetic engineering, stem cell research, and so on. The form of argument preferred by theologians had been to examine each technology in particular, and create condensed secular translations to discuss how it was or was not consistent with the myriad ends found in their traditions. They were interested in the technologies and the ends as a package, not only in the technologies themselves.

If theologians could not debate ends because they had been set by a common-morality principlist ethical system, what use were the theologians? In turns out there was no use for them, which was the beginning of the end of their influence. How had this specific method of common-morality principlism in the system of abstract knowledge become accepted as most appropriate by the jurisdiction-providers in research bioethics, health-care ethics consultation, and public policy bioethics, thus defeating the scientists and the theologians, and solidifying the jurisdictions of the bioethics profession?

The Structure and Content of Principlism

In my sociological approach, I do not assume that ethical systems such as principlism become influential because they are "the best" or "correct," but rather because the social conditions were right for the promoters of principlism to defeat those who had competing ideas. Being the "most coherent" ethical system, for example, is only an important factor in this competition if the people who give jurisdiction agree that "coherence" is the important standard, which is not always the case. The widespread belief in astrology should be enough to convince people that coherent idea systems do not automatically dominate.

The rise of principlism and the profession of bioethics was not because of its inherent excellence, but was rather the result of the rise of the government official as the jurisdiction-giver in the research bioethics and public policy bioethics task-spaces. In the health-care ethics consultation task-space, common-morality principlism later become dominant because it had the legitimacy of being endorsed by the government in research bioethics, it articulated with American law (critical for hospital administrators), it was easy to learn for the very part-time bioethicists who conducted health-care ethics consultation in small hospitals across the nation, and it fit well with the bureaucratic authority used in health-care institutions.

Principlism was appealing to jurisdiction-givers in the three jurisdictions because of the basic structure of the system and because of the content claim that the principles themselves were universally held by Americans. Let us start with the appeal of the basic structure or logic of principlism. All who have written about principlism can agree that to understand its dominance we must go back in history, perhaps to the Nuremberg trials after World War II. I propose that, to understand the appeal of principlism, and thus how the bioethics profession gained jurisdictions with it, we must go back much further, to 1494, when the first textbook for double-entry bookkeeping was written. This form of bookkeeping is the tabulation that anyone who uses a budget is familiar with: What are our costs for the next year? what is our income? And, more specifically; are the costs associated with this component of the business generating returns that justify the costs? This process is so taken-for-granted it is hard to imagine an alternative. Before the invention of this system, however, accounts from businesses were basically a "rambling story with numbers" that served to "assist the memory of the businessman," but not help with evaluation of the businessman's actions (Carruthers and Espeland 1991:40). For example, an account from the early fourteenth-century England stated:

> Account of Maurice Hunter and Fynlay Sutor, balies of the burgh of Stivelyn, given up at Dunbretan on the twenty-fifth day of January, . . . of the fermes of the said burgh for the two terms of this account. They charge themselves with £. 36 received on the account of the fermes of the said burgh for the year of their account. Whereof, for their superexpenses made in the preceding account 40 s. 1 d halfpenny. And in the duties to the abbot of Cambuskyneth and Dunfermelyn, . . . during the time of the account, £. 23, 5 s. 4 d. And to the Friars Preachers of Strivelyn. . . . (Carruthers and Espeland 1991:40).

The fifteenth century emergence of double-entry bookkeeping was a major innovation in economic history. Two changes in the accounts system also transformed it into a procedure that allowed for calculability, efficiency, and predictability in human action, paving the way for modern capitalism. The first change was that the new system was a means of discarding information deemed to be extraneous to the decision making. After all, does it matter to the calculation of profit that Hunter and Sutor lived in the burgh of Stivelyn? This could be put in an address book. The new accounting just had numbers, with all extraneous information removed.

The second change was that these numbers took on a new degree of calculability. Instead of there being proceeds on one list (the "rambling" account above) and costs on another, these two were translated into a common metric called "profit," making an evaluation of each action much more precise. With the previous, rambling narrative style of bookkeeping, owners could not readily determine whether an action (such as delivering to the abbot) was efficient at maximizing their end (profit). With the accounting that combined information about the costs and proceeds for dealings with the abbot, the efficacy of selling to him could be calculated.

The relevance of fifteenth-century bookkeepers to my argument is that a similar evolution in ideas has happened in bioethical debate and that revealing the similarity lets us tap into a long history of scholarship on these types of transformations. The previous babel of information formerly thought to be relevant to an ethical decision in the first two eras when scientists debated the theologians was whittled down to a much more manageable level through the use of pre-set principles, and the principles gave us a commensurable unit—akin to "profit" in bookkeeping—that also allowed for much simpler decisions.

Was there an era in bioethical debate equivalent to the "rambling narrative" style of bookkeeping? Yes—the two previous eras described in the last chapter. K. Danner Clouser describes medical ethics in the 1960s as "a mixture of religion, whimsy, exhortation, legal precedents, various traditions, philosophies of life, miscellaneous moral rules, and epithets" (Clouser 1993:S10). More generously, in a situation where anyone could come to the debate and provide a condensed translation of their ends, the resulting debate would have seemed quite disorderly to our eyes. With a disorderly system, how an ethical decision would be made was not calculable and predictable to anyone but the person making the decision, a point to which I will return below.

The logic of principlism does in fact offer the lure of calculability and predictability not offered by the jumble described by Clouser. This calculability and predictability can be summarized by the notion of *commensuration*. Commensuration is a method of "measuring different properties normally represented by different units with a single, common standard or unit" (Espeland 1998:24; Espeland and Stevens 1998:313–31). Philosophers will immediately recognize *utility* as one such commensurable metric. Scientists will recognize *risk/benefit analysis*, which translates all of the information of a situation into a universal commensurable metric of pleasure or pain. And all of us of course recognize *money*, the most common commensurable metric of all, where all sorts of objects and services can be put on one metric of value. Commensuration is essentially a method for discarding information in order to make decision making easier by ignoring aspects of the problem that cannot be translated to the common metric (Espeland 1998:25).

Principlism is a form of commensuration, although not as pure a form as money or utility, and not as commensurable as some critics would like.[9] If money or utility represents one commensurable scale, the principles as articulated by Beauchamp and Childress represent four metrics, with no agreed-upon method of deciding what to do when the metrics on the four scales point in different directions. In Veatch's summary, many "principled approaches . . . do not provide anything more than an intuitive balancing of conflicting appeals based on the judgement of the decision-maker" (Veatch 2007:43).

Yet, despite there being four principles and not one in Beauchamp and Childress' version, the principles are a system of commensuration nonetheless. They are a method taking the complexity of the multiple values held by the public and transforming this information into four scales by discarding information that resists transformation. To see the principles as commensuration, we can ask: Why are there four principles in the Beauchamp and Childress' system and not ten or perhaps twenty? Why did a member of the National Commission complain that there were "too many principles" in an early draft of the Belmont Report (there were seven), and that the list was not "crisp enough" (Jonsen 1998:103)? The answer is that the principles were created to enhance calculability or, in more common language, to simplify bioethical decision-making. For example, Beauchamp said that principles "provide frameworks of general guidelines that condensed morality to its central elements and gave people from diverse fields an easily grasped set of moral standards" (Beauchamp 1995:181).

This calculability or simplicity is first gained by discarding information about deeper epistemological or theoretical commitments. With Beauchamp, a professed "rule-utilitarian," and Childress, a professed "rule deontologist," this common metric of principles allowed for ethical decision-making they could both agree to, despite the massive amount of information about their ethical inclinations represented by the phrases "rule-utilitarian" and "rule-deontologist." They found that "many forms of rule utilitarianism and rule deontology lead to identical rules and actions." Yet, "rule-utilitarian" must provide some information about how to make a decision or the authors would no longer need such labels for themselves. Decision-making, despite long-standing differences between utilitarians and deontologists, can therefore be more efficiently calculated with the principles Jonsen called "the common coin of moral discourse" (Jonsen 1998:332–33).

Principlism as Transmutation

This simplification through commensuration made principlism extremely attractive to the new jurisdiction-givers for reasons I will discuss below. It is, however, a particular type of simplification. Principlism does not claim to engage in condensed translation, where a societal group's particular values or ends are translated without bias into the four principles. Rather, the claim is that since the four principles are all that are universally shared by the public, details of the values that cannot be pressed into the principles should be discarded.[10] This is *transmutation*, where the particularities are stated in the language of the principles as not necessarily accurate translations. For example, usually some of the concerns of religious groups can be stated using the principles, but not necessarily their core concerns, and then their core concerns are discarded for not being universally held. To see this simplifying commensuration process at work, I will show examples of transmutation from two federal bioethics commissions.

Consider the process that resulted in the report on human genetic engineering titled *Splicing Life* by a public policy bioethics entity, the President's Commission, of the early 1980s (President's Commission for the Study of Ethical Problems in Medicine and Biomedical and Behavioral Research 1983b). This process started when three religious leaders wrote to President Jimmy Carter in 1980, stating among their many claims that the evolving genetic technologies of the time would allow people to "play God" (Evans 2002:Ch. 4). The commission spent a very large amount of time on this phrase, and on the religious claims in general. As a religious-sounding phrase, "playing God" does not seem universal. Suffice it to say, they were confused, because not only did this phrase seem to have multiple meanings in the different religious traditions, it had seemed to evoke many claims simultaneously, and was thought to be vague.

From the perspective I am forwarding here, *vagueness* is simply another way of saying that the phrase contains far too much information. The phrase may have made sense to theologians, but not to bioethicists, so it needed to not only be "commensurated" (simplified), but transmuted into values or principles the bioethicists thought were universal. The commissioners thought they saw multiple concerns wrapped in the phrase: from concerns about creating new life forms, to fear of human knowledge, to ecological disaster.

How can one integrate all of these different perspectives? The staff did what they had to do to make a coherent report that tried to come to some conclusions: the claims were transmuted into the commensurable scale of principlism. They used the parts of principlism that seemed the most applicable and acceptable—risks and benefits (the principles of beneficence and non-maleficence)–and found various methods of discounting, putting off for later discussion, or "debunking" claims that could not be transmuted into these two established principles.

The analysis in the report begins by stating that "[a]lthough it does not have a specific religious meaning, the objection to scientists 'playing God' . . . appears to the Commission [to convey] several rather different ideas, some describing the power of gene splicing itself and some relating merely to its consequences." Note that there is no way to compare these competing claims about "gene splicing itself" without some overarching system of evaluation or metric. So therefore, in the report, claims about the technology "itself" were first "clarified," or, in the language of one of the people involved with the commission, "debunked" (Evans 2002:121).

After discrediting these claims—those difficult to transmute to the common metric of principlism—the commission turned to the two components of "playing God" that it felt deserved "serious consideration" (p. 57). The first is that since created life forms could reproduce, the possibility of "self-perpetuating mistakes" is a concern, but "the point is not that crossing species lines is inherently wrong, but that it may have *undesirable consequences* . . ." (my emphasis, p. 57). That is, it could violate the principle of non-maleficence.

The other "serious" objection in the phrase "playing God" is to human-animal hybrids, which reflects "the concern that human beings lack the God-like knowledge and wisdom required for the exercise of these God-like powers" (p. 58). It is pointed out that it is a legitimate problem that we may lack the scientific knowledge to avoid negative consequences. But, once again, this is not actually a prohibition because, "if this is the rational kernel of the admonition against playing God, then the use of gene splicing technology is not claimed to be wrong as such but wrong because of its potential consequences" (p. 58). The conclusion is that we must have more scientific data before we engage in creating human-animal hybrids, so that we know what the consequences are. That is, the research must go on so that we can weigh the risks and benefits— non-maleficence and beneficence.

In the final section of the report, possible outcomes of genetic engineering are discussed in light of their potential risks and benefits. The chapter concludes with the Commission stating that they "could find no ground for concluding that any current or planned forms of genetic engineering, whether using human or nonhuman material, are intrinsically wrong or irreligious per se" (p. 77). Principlism had created a language that could be used to discard enough information through transmutation to bring order to this difficult problem, and restate it using fixed common-morality principles.

Perhaps this was actually a condensed translation. That is, are the concerns of the theologians restated in the language of common-morality principlism accurate, albeit less precise, versions of what they were claiming, or were the concerns transmuted by focusing only on a subset of their claims? Not so, according to theologian Allen Verhey. Although the Commission deserved credit for trying to made sense of the phrase, he said, "the phrase does not so much state a principle as invoke a perspective on the world." It is not so much an argument to be dissected, but a way of referring to a series of arguments and method of decision-making typically used by theologians—a "fundamental perspective" (Verhey 1995:348, 350, 356). Summarizing these "fundamental perspectives" as "risks and benefits" surely leaves what others have called a specific "theological remainder," or, to put it put differently, results in information lost in the striving for a commensurable decision-making metric (Hanson 1999). The Commission engaged in transmutation, not translation.

The same type of transmutation can be seen fifteen years later in another government ethics commission where the bioethicists' system of abstract knowledge was in use—the National Bioethics Advisory Commission. In historian of science J. Benjamin Hurlbut's analysis, this commission's "approach reflected the procedural and principlist elements of professional bioethics" (Hurlbut 2010:186). Consistent with the bioethicists' system of abstract knowledge wherein they claim to be representing the public's values in the public policy bioethics jurisdiction, they wrote that "the construction of public policy on morally controversial matters should involve a 'search for significant points of convergence between one's own understandings and those of citizens whose positions, taken in their more comprehensive forms, one must reject'" (Hurlbut 2010:188). This means that only claims based on principles that are universally shared are legitimate. "The role of the public bioethics body, as [the Commission] saw it, was to translate religious reasons into a secular, ideologically neutral, normative idiom that could, as far as possible, unify the moral pluralism of the American public" (Hurlbut 2010:189). (While Hurlbut uses the term *translation*, by my terminology he is describing transmutation.)

The result was that "public policy should incorporate only those positions that can be translated into generic, common principles" (Hurlbut 2010:190). Therefore, transmutation to principlism allows the bioethics profession to be inclusive of all Americans by taking account of their reasons, while simultaneously transmuting reasons into preexisting principles. This makes them easily actionable by unelected officials because the bioethicists' claims are portrayed as translations of everyone's values into universal values. Like the President's Commission of the early 1980s, this was transmutation, not condensed translation. Hurlbut concludes that "certain commissioners repeatedly commented on the difficulties of translating the [religious] to the [ethical.] Translation came to be a gatekeeping device: if commissioners could not come up with what they thought was a reasonable translation of a theological claim, they excluded it" (Hurlbut 2010:190).

Discarding of information and transmutation to ostensibly universally held principles is not considered a flaw by the bioethics profession. Indeed, this transmutation to a common metric in order to allow simplified ethical decision-making in a pluralistic society is often considered *the* achievement of the bioethics profession. What, then, does this description of principlism as transmutation and information-discarding get us? It is now easier to understand why common-morality principlism allowed the bioethics profession to gain the research bioethics, health-care ethics consultation, and public policy bioethics jurisdictions. It is also easier to understand why (I will later argue) a form of common-morality principlism needs to still be used in these jurisdictions.

The Preference for Common Morality Among Jurisdiction-Givers

The bureaucratic state became the jurisdiction-provider for research bioethics and public policy bioethics. Beyond principlism's logic or structure, its substantive-content claim to represent the common morality obviously made it attractive to government officials, and this appeal is acknowledged by its designers. Beauchamp and Childress, in arguing against classical forms of justification from philosophy, write that: "[i]f we could be confident that some abstract moral theory was a better source for codes and policies than the common morality, we could work constructively on practical and policy questions by progressively specifying the norms of that theory. At present, we have no such theory." They add that they "cannot reasonably expect that an inherently contestable moral theory will be better for practical decision-making and policy development than the morality that serves as our common heritage" (Beauchamp and Childress 2009:388–89).

With common morality, the morals are claimed to be the morals of everyone. The unelected official is simply engaged in the rule-like following of the values of the people, and it would then be less controversial. I can imagine nothing that would outrage the American public more than being told that an unelected government official had decided what values the public would want to be pursued through medical research.

The structure or logic of principlism, independent of its content, also provides an advantage compared to other professions' arguments, in a context where the state is the jurisdiction-provider. It is here that the relevance of fifteenth-century bookkeeping is found. The literature on the rise of these commensurable, calculable decision systems points to the state as one of the foremost proponents. Of course, the birth of common-morality principlism itself is twinned with the advent of state intervention in ethics. Warren Reich, in discussing the early days of the Kennedy Institute, which later was the birthplace of principlism, says that, in the early 1970s, "there was a political urgency to many of the biomedical issues," and that "the media craved the biomedical controversies and federal and state policymakers wanted answers." Principlism was "evidently found more congenial to the educational and policymaking purposes being pursued" than what he saw as its competitor.[11] It was "open to a broad range of concepts and arguments, in particular those that favored clarification in the public forum of policymaking." Reich goes on to describe how the founder of the Kennedy Institute "marshaled hitherto untapped federal and private funding" and "fostered the need for medical bioethics in the government agencies."[12] Jonsen later concluded that the principles, which had become part of public law, had "met the need of public-policy makers for a clear and simple statement of the ethical basis for regulation of research" (Jonsen 1994:xvi).

It is critical to ask: Why did government policy makers need a "clear and simple statement of the ethical basis of research?" To put it in the terms used in this chapter, why did policy makers need a commensurable ethical scale that discarded information? There are two primary reasons. First, government authority in Western liberal democracies such as the United States needs to be transparent to the citizens. Second, this government is bureaucratic.

In liberal democracies, decision-making must be transparent. Unlike decrees coming from the subjective perspective of the European sovereign, the American political system was partly founded "on the idea that politics is transparent, that political agents, political actions, and political power can be viewed" (Ezrahi 1990:69). The surface manifestation of this impulse is that government decision-making proceedings—like bioethics commissions—have open meetings, allowing the public to view the decision-making process undertaken on its behalf by its elected officials (and appointed officials, like commissioners). The more subtle manifestation of the need for transparency is that government decision-making tends to use methods that purport to be objectively transparent.

Historian Theodore Porter explains the popularity of commensurable scales in government decision-making, such as cost–benefit analysis, to be the result of government officials needing to appear to not really be exercising their own judgement, but following transparent and objective laws or rules. As he puts it, in other countries government officials are "trusted to exercise judgment wisely and fairly. In the United States, they are expected to follow rules" (Porter 1995:195). This is because, simply, it is part of the U.S. political culture to not trust authority, especially government authority, and the authority of bureaucrats in particular. A complex decision means that we would have to trust the judgement of the government functionary, because they cannot readily explain how they reached their judgement. In the words of one analyst, "in a country where mistrust of government is rife, the temptation to substitute supposedly impersonal calculation for personal, responsible decisions . . . cannot but be exceedingly strong."[13]

In contrast to the United States, "in some societies the right of government officials to make decisions is taken for granted. People may disagree about the substance of the decision but they do not question the authority behind it" (Wilson 1989:303). Another study finds that compared to the distrust of experts in the United States, the "more insulated regulatory processes of both Britain and

Germany historically depended on greater trust in expertise." In the United Kingdom, objective knowledge is pursued "through consultation among persons whose capacity to discern the truth is regarded as privileged" (Jasanoff 2005:262, 266).

If Americans do not trust government officials to exercise their discretion over where to build a dam (one of Porter's examples), they certainly do not trust the government to make what are construed as moral decisions. Therefore, an Institutional Review Board in the research bioethics task-space that is indirectly representing the government cannot simply approve of research because they "think" that it is ethical, but must rather "show" or, better yet, "prove" with objective, transparent methods, that the research is ethical (Ezrahi 1990:Ch. 3). They must show their reasoning in a manner that the public can judge.[14] Weighing and balancing pre-set principles such as beneficence and non-maleficence (risks and benefits)—notice the simple decision-making rule—purports to be more transparent. Like the allure of cost–benefit analysis, the public can feel that it understands the decision being made on its behalf, giving the decision legitimacy.

Again, compare this to Europe. In the United Kingdom, the Human Fertilisation and Embryology Authority determines which genetic diseases are serious enough to warrant genetic intervention. This sort of setting of societal values or purposes about what a "serious" disease is by an unelected government body would be unlikely to happen in the United States, where the refrain "policies would be set by those bureaucrats in Washington" is considered to be a convincing argument against universal health care.

The second reason for the allure of the logic of principlism is the fact that the parts of the government that are supposed to protect us ethically are bureaucracies. Bureaucracies evolved to control larger and larger institutions, and part of this ability to control far-flung activities is to create standardized rules (Perrow 1986:Ch. 1; Weber 1968:220–23). Standardized rules, even in ethics, are desirable from a bureaucratic perspective.

Consider the IRB system, which, in classic bureaucratic form, has "guidelines" which are to be used by recipients of federally funded research involving human experimentation. Each institution must set up a committee to make ethical decisions for the government, and the government mandates that certain ethical principles be used and records which must be kept. Imagine the bureaucratic chaos if each IRB were able to determine its own principles. The key problem would be that the NIH would not be able to demonstrate to its congressional overseers that proper ethics were actually in use.

The bureaucracy has become even more important since the 1960s. Not only is there the Office for the Protection from Research Risks that supervises the IRBs in the research bioethics task-space, but there have been ethics committees spread throughout the federal bureaucracy in the public policy bioethics task-space, such as the Recombinant DNA Advisory Committee. Each of these must demonstrate that it is making transparent decisions, and common-morality principlism is useful for this.

Bureaucracy does not only exist in the government, of course. David Rothman notes that the era of the rise of bioethics and common-morality principlism was also the era of the decline of trust in physicians (Rothman 1991). If we do not know our physicians, thanks to the rise of bureaucracies such as managed care, group practices, as well as increasing residential mobility, the argument goes, we do not know their values, either. At this point, we turn to observable decision-making systems like principlism in order to create trust.

This explains part of the attractiveness of principlism to the bureaucratized jurisdiction-providers in health-care ethics consultation. Moreover, as touted by its proponents, due to its simplicity, principlism is easy to learn for the very part-time bioethicists who engage in this task. A practicing nurse who engages in three ethics consults a year (a not-uncommon rate: see Fox, Myers and Pearlman 2007) does not need to earn a doctorate in bioethics, but can read a fairly straightforward textbook about the four principles.[15] In sum, the rise of the bureaucratic state (and the bureaucratic health-care organization) as jurisdiction-givers for (and consumers of) ethics in three of the four jurisdictions has contributed to a preference for the method of common-morality principlism used in the system of abstract knowledge of the bioethics profession. The bioethics profession won all three jurisdictions.

The Growing Dominance of Common-Morality Principlism in the Bioethics Profession's Jurisdictions

The first jurisdictional success of the bioethics profession was in research bioethics, where common-morality principlism had become institutionalized. Bioethics expanded to health-care ethics consultation, which is also dominated by principlism (Bosk 2010). In the words of one bioethicist, principlism "grew from the principles underlying the conduct of research into the basic principles of bioethics" (Jonsen 1998:104).

As the jurisdictions of the bioethics profession grew in importance, and as principlism became the ethical system that was required by law to be used in human experimentation throughout the country, more and more people learned this system. Institutional Review Boards at institutions that receive federal research money use principlism to make their decisions, essentially spreading the principlist system farther and farther.

Many observers have noted the absolute dominance of the principlist system embodied in Beauchamp's and Childress's textbook, which Hoffmaster calls "the Bible of academic medical ethics" (1991:219). Similarly, Dubose claims that this one book has more than anything else "shaped the teaching and practice of biomedical ethics in this country . . . [becoming] a standard text in courses and a virtual bible to some practitioners." The ethical framework provided by the book "shapes much of the discussion and debate about particular bioethical issues and policy, whether in the academy, the literature, the public forum or the clinic" (DuBose, Hamel and O'Connell 1994:1). The institutionalization of this form of argumentation for human experimentation and increasingly for other problems was so strong that one set of critics begin their essay with the mocking claim that "throughout the land, arising from the throngs of converts to bioethics awareness, there can be heard a mantra '... beneficence ... autonomy ... justice. ...'" (Clouser, K. Danner and Gert 1990:219). Fox and Swazey have recently claimed that the approach in the book "has been so widely disseminated across national boundaries that it has become a kind of bioethical lingua franca" (Fox and Swazey 2008:216). Others have shown how it is being imported wholesale into non-Western countries (DeVries, Rott and Paruchuri 2011). The influential textbook created specifically for health-care ethics consultation, *Clinical Ethics: A Practical Approach to Ethical Decisions in Clinical Medicine*, now in its sixth edition, states that "there is general agreement that modern medical ethics depends on a small group of moral principles: respect for the autonomy of patients, beneficence, non-maleficence, and justice" (Jonsen, Siegler and Winslade 2006:2). These principles are so undebatable that the book has a four-fold table with the principles as headings in each box, listing questions the consulting ethicist should ask at the bedside (Jonsen, Siegler and Winslade 2006:11). A copy of this table on card stock is included at the end of the book so that it can be torn out and put in your pocket when walking around the hospital. Similarly, *The Handbook for Health Care Ethics Committees*, designed to train members of hospital ethics committees, writes that the "core ethical principles that support the therapeutic relationship and give rise to clinical obligations include respecting patient autonomy ... beneficence ... nonmaleficence ... [and] distributive justice." For more details the authors suggest consulting the dominant description of common-morality principlism written by Beauchamp and Childress (Post, Blustein and Dubler 2007: 15, 17).[16]

While principlism has been strongest in research bioethics, health-care ethics consultation, and public policy bioethics, it has also made serious inroads into cultural bioethics, as gatekeepers in the broader public sphere—like newspaper reporters and editors—turn to bioethicists for commentary on what the public should think about new developments in science and medicine. In an analysis of media discourse in the United States and the United Kingdom concerning "therapeutic cloning," sociologist Eric Jensen compares the prevalence of the form of argumentation used in eras one and two (debates about ends) with the form of argumentation in era three (debates using Beauchamp and Childress' principlist system). He concludes that "the overall trend clearly favours the four principles in both the American and British press samples" (Jensen 2008:196). However, this was not monolithic, and particularly in the United States, some participants continued to use the old form of argumentation in cultural bioethics, particularly in the 2001–2006 articles in his sample (Jensen 2008:196), which coincide with the rise of the crisis in the bioethics profession.

Along with the gaining of jurisdiction over research bioethics and health-care ethics consultation, the bioethics profession also saw the task-space of public policy bioethics expand. At first there was only one issue in public policy bioethics: human experimentation. Soon, public policy bioethics addressed all issues in science and medicine. This is bluntly indicated by the difference in the titles of the first and second government ethics commissions. The first, the "National Commission" was "for the Protection of Human Subjects of Biomedical and Behavioral Research." The second, the "President's Commission" was "for the Study of Ethical Problems in Medicine and Biomedical and Behavioral Research." Medicine and biomedical and behavioral "research" suggests a much more expansive task than "protection of human subjects," and the reports issued by the latter commission reflected this expansiveness.

The End of the Theological Challenge in Three Jurisdictions

To return to our historical narrative, the early institutionalization of common-morality principlism concerned some of the original advocates of broader bioethical debates that would include theologians, especially as common-morality principlism came to be used in cultural bioethics. As early as 1982, Daniel Callahan was warning about the new hegemony in ethical thinking in these debates. Calling this new hegemony "some kind of ultimate moral big bang theory" or an "'engineering model' of applied ethics," he bemoaned the emphasis on narrow forms of argumentation like principlism. The broader approach that he had championed in the early days of the field had "the distinct advantage of leaving the way open for the insights of religion, of cultural observation and social analysis . . . and of concepts of human dignity and purpose that had a wider scope than mere autonomy." Opposing the creation of a separate profession of bioethics with its own system of abstract knowledge, he hoped that "the other disciplines that are a part of applied ethics, will . . . shout and scream" when they detect the "diversion from what was intended to be a richer agenda" (Callahan 1982:4). That is, it was not only theologians who were turned off by the newly required system of abstract knowledge, but anyone interested in debating ends, such as sociologists and Continental philosophers who were more abstract and uninterested in mid-range principles.

There were of course theologians who complained and resisted their jurisdictional defeat, continuing to engage in either explicit or implicit condensed translations of theological ends. Ramsey later purportedly "refused to let the more theological parts of [his 1978] *Ethics at the Edges of Life* be edited out, explicitly to rebut the criticism that *The Patient as Person* was insufficiently theological" (Hauerwas 1996:66). However, in general, as common-morality principlism grew, theologians (and others) lost interest in the debates in research bioethics, health-care ethics consultation, and public policy bioethics, abandoning attempts at jurisdiction. As Gustafson has written, "it is not easy to give a clearly theological answer to a question that is formulated so that there are no theological aspects to it" (Gustafson 1978:387). It is important to note that this was not a conspiracy. There was no meeting at which the bioethicists said "how do we get these theologians out of the debate?" Rather, it was a gradual process that primarily worked through cohort replacement, not a strong change in the way any one person debated these issues. Primarily, the debate changed as people who wanted to debate the ends to pursue through technology—or who wanted to discuss a plethora of ends more generally—decided not to enter bioethical debate, and those who wanted to speak about these issues and who were already in the debate left for greener pastures or retired.

Theology had defended its jurisdiction from scientists, but had subsequently lost the jurisdictional challenge to the bioethics profession. By the late 1990s, when an explicitly theological voice did make an appearance in public policy bioethics, participants questioned the legitimacy of including this voice, even if secular translations were offered. An example of this was the hearings in the late 1990s on human cloning. The National Bioethics Advisory Commission found itself in a swirl of controversy when a Scottish research team announced that they had cloned a sheep, and President Clinton gave this Commission a very short time to come to an ethical conclusion. A panel of theologians was invited to the hearing, and some of them did indeed make very theological statements—including a Ramseyesque statement by one of Ramsey's former students.

Although invited to speak, the input of the theologians was registered but did not seem to have any impact on the conclusions. A consultant to the Commission who wrote a paper on religious perspectives on cloning would later claim that "the contributions of the religious perspectives were deemed politically important and ethically insignificant" (Campbell 1997).

There were even complaints about the involvement of theologians at all. An article by three bioethicists critiquing a report—two of whom are extremely influential in the field—complained that "the rationale for considering explicitly religious perspectives, in a political system governed by a core commitment to the separation of church and state and marked by pervasive pluralism, receives scant attention in the report. It fails to clarify why or how religious views and voices could or should shape public policy with respect to cloning" (Miller, Caplan and Fletcher 1998:265). Jurisdiction of the bioethics profession with its common-morality system of abstract knowledge was increasingly secure. By the end of the century, there remained some theologians who are as theological in their writing as such writing ever was, but they were largely competing in the final contested jurisdictional space of cultural bioethics.

Some scholars, particularly the card-carrying members of the theological remnant, have discussed this history. They have talked about how the "renaissance of medical ethics" was quickly followed by its "enlightenment," where "interest in religious traditions moved from the center to the margins of scholarly attention" (Verhey and Lammers 1993:3). Reasons for the "enlightenment" remain unexamined, except through reference to recognition of the pluralism of American society. I have tried to sketch the more detailed causes of the "enlightenment" here.

Over the past two chapters, I have told this history in three stages, while most observers of the secularization of bioethics simply talk about "the religious time" and "the irreligious time." I have described three overlapping phases: First, when theologians, challenged by scientists who seemed to be attempting to determine the meaning and purpose of humanity through science, entered these debates using explicit condensed translations of theological ends. This attempt at explicit translation was extremely short-lived. For a number of reasons having to do with the audience of the theologians and the nature of the theological profession itself, theologians during what I call the second period turned to secular condensed translations without explicit connection to the original religious ends. This debate was a debate about ends—with each particularistic group using its own tradition to determine ends, there were many to debate. Even this debate about the proper ends to pursue was not to last, as the rise of government and bureaucratic jurisdiction-givers required a simple, transparent universal system of ends to pursue that theologians were uninterested in. Principlism created a set of predetermined ends, portrayed as universally held by the people. The bioethics profession, largely using its common-morality principlism method in its system of abstract knowledge, now had solid jurisdiction over research bioethics and health-care ethics consultation. It had a fairly solid jurisdiction over public policy bioethics. Bioethicists were more and more found in the cultural bioethics debate as well, becoming the authoritative profession for insights about the ethics of science and medicine. However, the bioethics profession's jurisdiction over public policy bioethics was not as solid as it may have originally appeared.

Notes

1. In Stark (2012: 154).

2. The previous three paragraphs are informed by Stark (2012).

3. My emphasis. See Edwards and Sharpe (1971:89, 90).

4. Cited in Jonsen (1994:xiv).

5. According to historian of science J. Benjamin Hurlbut, another method of making the ethical claims articulate with the values of the general public that developed later in the public policy bioethics jurisdiction has been called "reasonable accommodation." This method is exemplified by its use in the Human Embryo Research Panel (HERP) of the mid-1990s. The panel was to ethically evaluate research on extracorporeal human embryos and report to the Advisory Committee to the Director of the National Institutes of Health, as the director needed to make decisions about using NIH money for embryo research (Hurlbut 2010:120)

> Great efforts were made to try to create a "neutral" ethical analysis. The Panel would not find the one true answer to what the embryo is, but rather to find the common ground among the "reasonable" claims that are held by the public. The panel

called this a "'pluralistic' approach," and "rather than adopt a single criterion such as genetic diploidy, sentience or self-concept, the pluralist approach avoided privileging any one criterion. It emphasized "a variety of distinct, intersecting, and mutually supporting considerations." In light of different views of the embryo in the public, the Panel wrote that "it is not the role of those who help form public policy to decide which of these views is correct. Instead, public policy represents an effort to arrive at a reasonable accommodation to diverse interests" (Hurlbut 2010:127–28).

If the "reasonable" arguments would be balanced, determining which arguments were "reasonable" was key. The Panel cited political theorist John Rawls to the effect that reasons must be understandable by all citizens. This eliminates those based on what Rawls called comprehensive perspectives, like religion. Hurlbut continues:

Guided by Rawls's notion of public reason, HERP set about to determine what (and whose) arguments should be included in the pluralist approach. In assuming a role as arbiter of public reason, the panel saw itself as judging moral arguments not on their merits but on their reasonableness. Arguments were given greater weight if the Panel imagined a reasonable public would find them convincing. The more arguments drew on premises held in common, the more weight they were given. [The chair of the Panel] argued that the Panel's task was to sort public reasons from nonpublic ones, and in so doing, stand in for an ideally democratic and ideally rational community of judgement (Hurlbut 2010:129).

So the panel challenged arguments that came from comprehensive perspectives. It privileged those that referred to scientific facts, because these were thought to be more widely accessible. "The Panel treated accounts that invoked scientific evidence as closer to public reasons— closer to the view from everywhere [on] which all reasonable minds would necessarily agree" (Hurlbut 2010:131). It is important to note that this is a particular type of common morality. The panel thought it would adjudicate between the different moralities when recommending public policy, but only those that could, using a particular version of liberal democratic theory, be expressed in the public sphere. This method has not been extensively used in the public policy bioethics jurisdiction.

A second approach to identifying the public's morality was taken up by this same panel. They looked to determine the common morality by seeing what the public actually did. For example, the widespread use of intrauterine devices, which result in the death of embryos, were thought of "as proxies for widespread moral intuitions about the moral status of the embryo" (Hurlbut 2010:132). This has remained a rarely used method of argument for bioethicists, probably because there were not too many analogies like this to be had. The point of reviewing the more minor methods is to see how bioethicists consider it a requirement of their jurisdictions to be forwarding the values of the general public.

6. While the Belmont Report talked about "respect for persons" through the lens of autonomy, scholars have noted that the subtle shift from the Belmont version to the Beauchamp and Childress version creates subtle differences in the conclusions one would reach. Theologians agree that by the time Ramsey's translation of covenant to respect for persons had been filtered through the Belmont Report and Beauchamp and Childress, the covenant part was gone, leaving "autonomy" as libertarianism (Lysaught 2004:678; Lebacqz 2005).

7. Robert Veatch has a similar view of the plasticity of principles, arguing that "other theories do not use the language of principles, but nevertheless present short general lists of normative moral criteria for morally right action, calling them duties (sometimes prima facie duties), rules or 'appeals'" (Veatch 2007:43). Similarly, John Harris sees "the four principles" as constituting "a useful 'checklist' approach to bioethics for those new to the field, and possibly for ethics committees without substantial ethical expertise . . . approaching new problems." He goes on to reject principles because they would "lead to sterility and uniformity of approach of a quite mind bogglingly boring kind" (Harris 2003:303).

8. While "principlism" generally refers to this four-principle system popularized by Beauchamp and Childress, there are many less influential but similar and competing systems in bioethics that share the same logic. For example, Robert Veatch identifies single-principle theories, like utilitarianism and libertarianism, that maximize the values of beneficence and autonomy, respectively. Two-principle theories include the "geometric method" of comparing benefits and harms, and Engelhardt's approach, which uses the principles of permission and beneficence. Other systems have five principles (Baruch Brody), six principles (W.D. Ross), seven principles (Veatch's own system) and ten principles (Bernard Gert) (Veatch 2007). For my purposes I will call

these all "principlism" because they are based on fixed principles that can be used for any bioethical issue. This obviously glosses over some differences in order to generalize. I will generally make reference to Beauchamp's and Childress's specific ethical system because it is far and away the most influential. Note, however, that not all of these alternative systems explicitly presume a common morality.

9. Readers may recognize this as the heart of the critique of principlism by K. Danner Clouser and Bernard Gert. Although I will not go into the details of their critique, what is most important for the discussion at hand is that the principles are not a "universal moral theory." More than one, or sometimes all, of the four principles may be applicable to any given case, and the principles provide no mechanism for adjudicating between them. Clouser and Gert believe strongly in the "unity of morality" and believe that "everyone must agree on the procedure to be used in deciding moral questions." See Clouser, K. Danner and Gert (1990:236).

10. In political-theory terms, principlism is John Rawls's public reason (Rawls 1993).

11. The competitor that Reich is discussing is the notion of bioethics as described by Van Rensselaer Potter.

12. Reich (1995:22, 23). Reich also clearly believes that the founder's personality had something to do with this as well.

13. Richard Hammond, in Theodore Porter, *Trust in Numbers: The Pursuit of Objectivity in Science and Public Life*, 195.

14. Indeed, the list of these principles can be found online in the IRB Guidebook, published by the Department of Health and Human Services. Available at http://www.hhs.gov/ohrp/archive/irb/irb_guidebook.htm.

15. The government itself has mandated that autonomy be one of the ethical principles in health-care ethics consultation, as court decisions have found that a patient has a right to determine their own health decision-making in decisions such as when to stop treatment (Bosk 2010:S137), so the use of principlism in health-care ethics consultation is perhaps over-determined.

16. Two other authors go as far as to say that "by establishing itself as the state-sanctioned authority for converting discussions of good and bad in American medical science into a common language and concepts, the bioethics of principlism achieved the status of an ascendant

political currency with global potential" (Salter and Salter 2007:561). Ebbesen and Pedersen, in the process of testing whether principlism really represents the common morality, conclude that the principlism of Beauchamp and Childress "is one of the most influential bioethical theories in the world" (Ebbesen and Pedersen 2007:36).

Others do not explain why principlism in particular rose to prominence within bioethics, but see it as the unifying discourse of bioethicists. For example, Dzur writes that "for scholars interested in ethics and medicine the *Belmont Report* and *Principles of Biomedical Ethics* represented an imaginary consensus on general rules, a common starting point for interpretation and reconstruction . . . to speak with one another, to collaborate, to critique productively, bioethicists required such an imaginary consensus" (Dzur 2002:192).

PART II

Contributions to the Jurisdictional Crisis

Chapter 3

The Rise of the Social-Movement Activists

The system of abstract knowledge of the bioethics profession is based on the idea that it is not using the values of the bioethicist, or of a subgroup of citizens, but the values of either those involved in a decision (health-care ethics consultation) or the general public (research bioethics and public policy bioethics). This worked extremely well in the 1970s and 1980s because the fit between this system of abstract knowledge and the jurisdiction-givers in the bureaucratic state was tight. As explained in Chapter 2, common-morality principlism in particular met the needs of the bureaucratic state, as well as other bureaucratic institutions, and the bioethics profession was rewarded with jurisdiction. Jurisdiction was rewarded as the jurisdiction-providers paid attention to bioethicists and not others.

The providers of jurisdiction have lately stopped buying the bio-ethical product, suggesting the fit is no longer so good. This is analo-gous to a situation where sick people no longer go to physicians and instead go to acupuncturists because they have lost faith in the phy-sicians' ability to heal their disease. The jurisdiction-providers in public policy bioethics are still the employees of the bureaucratic state (e.g., the director of NIH) and increasingly the elected officials who ultimately oversee the bureaucratic officials (e.g., members of Congress). However, the perspective of these jurisdiction-givers on bioethical issues has changed over the past 40 years, and they are increasingly selecting social-movement activists over bioethicists for the task of recommending ethical advice for policy.

The Changing Nature of the Jurisdiction-Givers

How could the idea of forwarding common morality through principlism or some other method be considered obviously true in one era and obviously not true in the next? It all depends upon who the audience is. Common-morality principlism was invented at a time when it could be imagined that there was a moral consensus among participants with power in the public sphere. However, the days where it could appear that there was a common morality among the elites in the public sphere concerning bioethical issues are gone, and this makes the jurisdictional crisis in bioethics all the more apparent and urgent.

The early years of bioethical debate are a nice example of an era when people could imagine a common morality on these issues. In Chapter 1, I described the mainline Protestantism of the 1950s as a religion that was very sure of itself, thinking it could speak for everyone in America, even those of different religions. I also discussed the growing religious pluralism in the public sphere and how this led to a decline in explicitly theological claims. But this growing pluralism in the public sphere was only among types of religious liberals. Whereas before there were only (liberal) mainline Protestants, later there were also liberal Jews and liberal Catholics. As sociologists have shown, the liberals in diverse traditions have more in common with each other than do the liberals and conservatives within one tradition (Wuthnow 1988).

Why no fundamentalists or evangelicals? They were still in retreat from the world after their fights with the mainline Protestants in the 1920s. Why no traditionalist Catholics? It is clear from debates within Vatican II that the type of Catholics acceptable to the mainline establishment were the liberals (Wilde 2007). Since it was only religious liberals who participated in the elite public sphere, claiming there was a common morality might have seemed plausible in that all of these religious traditions had drunk deeply from the well of Enlightenment rationality. The early theologians in the debate reflected the liberal religious nature of public-sphere elites. Moreover, I am not aware of any fundamentalists, evangelicals, or traditionalist Catholics who were involved during those early years of bioethical debate.[1] Perhaps half of the population of the United States were religiously unrepresented in bioethical debates.

After the invention of principlism, and in the same period that bioethical debates were becoming more secular because the liberal theologians started moving away from them (period 3), evangelicals and fundamentalists decided to reenter public life, joining traditionalist Catholics who were already active in the public sphere on issues like abortion. This is the now-familiar story of the post-1979 emergence of the "religious right" in American politics (Wuthnow 1988; Moen 1992).

Mainline Protestants have influence on public life, *not* through the ballot box, nor through political activism, nor grassroots organizing, but rather through elite influence (Wuthnow and Evans 2002). They have influence by being the establishment, and bioethical debate was an establishment activity, consisting of some academics and a few government commissions making recommendations about what was ethical. The general public was not deeply involved. Indeed, the whole point of the public policy bioethics was to shape that debate in such a way that the public did not need to get involved, since bioethicists were representing the public's values.

It should therefore be no surprise that when conservative Protestants in the religious right reentered the public sphere, they originally decided that they could not influence the world through the establishment activity of the liberal Protestants, like public policy bioethics, but instead would influence the world by social-movement organizing and influencing elections. Not only was this an accurate assessment of their constraints, it fit quite well with one of the core beliefs of evangelicals, which is that they are a beleaguered minority that is oppressed by the powers that be (Smith 1998).

What is important for our purposes is that slowly, over time, the religious right did two things. First, it built up a large machinery for influencing public policy, including think tanks and social-movement organizations such as the Christian Coalition, Concerned Women for America, and Focus on the Family. Second, it became a core constituent of, or took over—depending on one's view—the national Republican Party (Wilcox 2009), and therefore grained great influence over elected officials.

Bioethical debates remained largely under the radar of the religious conservatives and the religious right in the late 1970s and early 1980s. Early bioethical debates about mind control, human experimentation, human genetic engineering, psychosurgery, and the like were just not central to their concerns, and they did not pay attention to the ethical advice government officials were receiving.

After that point, there was growing attention from elite religious conservatives to public policy bioethics, partially due to attention given to a number of government ethics commissions that discussed embryos. Embryo research was more and more desired by scientists as it increasingly seemed that embryonic stem cells might have some therapeutic use. Bioethical debate increasingly had actual influence on what happened in the world, making it more important to fight over (Caplan 2005:13).

Did religious conservatives think they should have their young people get doctoral degrees in bioethics and get involved with the bioethics profession? Of course not. Bioethical debate as an elite institution was still closed to these perspectives, because the ethical system these religious conservatives wanted to use was not in favor in bioethical debate. Many religious conservatives were not in favor of implicit *or* explicit translation, let alone transmutation. Since the mainstream in the debate does not accept their reasoning, they knew that they could not win through "reasoned arguments" with bioethicists or others in the debate. Indeed, their reasoning was the part of the argument that was shed with the transmutation. So, to have influence, they needed to act like a social movement. Luckily, they already had one, at least on some of these issues, which was the right-to-life movement and the machinery of the religious right more broadly. These movements brought great attention to any ethical policy recommendations that had to do with beginning- and end-of-life issues that were being proposed for government policy. Government officials could no longer ignore their perspective.

The Telling Case of Commissions Focused on Embryos

So, in the public sphere more broadly, social-movement activists in the religious right were articulating ethical claims, often concerning beginning- and end-of-life issues, that were distinct from those articulated by the bioethics profession. The history of bioethics commissions focused on embryos shows that the methods in the system of abstract knowledge of the bioethics profession were decreasingly accepted by the jurisdiction-givers in the government because of the rise of the religious right.

You can count the number of federal government ethics commissions in various ways, but I count eleven, beginning with the first: the National Commission for the Protection of Human Subjects of Biomedical and Behavioral Research, in 1974.[2] The commissions where the religious right was watching closely were contested and the ethical recommendations of the commissions unlikely to be implemented. Conservative dissatisfaction with the system of abstract knowledge used by the bioethicists in this jurisdiction mounted with time.

While the first bioethics commission dealt with research on fetuses, the first of the bioethics commissions to deal with embryos was the Ethics Advisory Board of the Department of Health, Education and Welfare (1978–1980), which was designed to advise the secretary of the department on "problematic protocols." It primarily worked on a report called "research involving human in vitro fertilization and embryo transfer."

Note that liberal theologians were still often on these commissions, particularly in the earlier years, as they could still promote their secular translations of implicitly theological ends as one of the diverse groups that could generate the common morality through consensus. In later years, when principlism became more institutionalized, theologians were less commonly on commissions.

What was interesting for my purposes is that the 1978 Commission came up with a recommendation to allow embryo research up to 14 days after fertilization. Note that this recommendation was endorsed by a Catholic theologian on the Commission after he was persuaded by another Catholic theologian who testified, as official Catholic views of early embryos were still in flux during this era (Banchoff 2011:37-40).

The public comment period following the release of the report produced nearly 13,000 letters, all but 300 opposing IVF research, and many of these letters were the result of organized protests of "religious groups" (Green 2001:2). In this era these would have been traditionalist Roman Catholics and the right-to-life social movement organizations the Catholic Church either created or worked with. This suggested that conservative religious people did not accept the bioethicists' work.

The Commission made its recommendations to the head of Department of Health, Education and Welfare in May of 1979, but that head left later that year before acting on it. The new director was very busy, and the report fell by the wayside. Later, the Ethics Advisory Board's budget was folded into the budget for the new President's Commission that would begin at this time (Hurlbut 2010:80). The Ethics Advisory Board died a quiet death.

During the 1980s a number of groups made calls for the reconstitution of the Ethics Advisory Board so that embryo research could be funded by the government. Calls came from the American Fertility Society, the National Advisory Child Health and Human Development Council, and the American Association for the Advancement of Science (Hurlbut 2010:109). At a congressional hearing, a representative of the US Conference of Catholic Bishops argued, in Hurlbut's words, "that the purpose of a reconstituted [Ethics Advisory Board] would be to provide unilateral approval of IVF experimentation without any mechanism for democratic intervention" (Hurlbut 2010:112). Clearly, the Catholic bishops did not believe that the bioethics methods used by the Ethics Advisory Board would result in democratic decisions, and thought that it would say "yes" to the desires of scientists.

In an exchange with an advocate of reconstituting the Board, Republican representative Dennis Hastert proclaimed, "so actually we have a board of people who are quote unquote 'experts' . . . and they're actually making moral decisions from a wide spectrum—even at this table we have quite a divergent view of what's right and wrong—but somebody in the place of the legislator . . . would be making those decisions on whether this in vitro fertilization . . . for the purpose of experimentation should take place or should not take place" (in Hurlbut 2010: 113). Hastert clearly did not accept the Ethics Advisory Board's recommendations as neutral. Hurlbut concludes that "behind these various characterizations of the EAB was a disagreement over the democratic role of the ethics body that became even more pronounced as subsequent ethics bodies were formed in the 1990s and 2000s" (Hurlbut 2010:113). Bioethicist Ronald Green concludes that the de facto moratorium on embryo research of the Reagan and George H. W. Bush years, resulting from the lack of an Ethics Advisory Board, "despite efforts to end it by various NIH and HHS administrators . . . was maintained because both administrations were aligned with 'right to life' constituencies that opposed any manipulations of human embryos" (Green 2001:3).

In 1985, Congress authorized the creation of a biomedical ethics board made up of six representatives and six senators evenly split between the two parties, who would appoint a biomedical ethics advisory committee. These entities were to make a report on human genetic engineering and the federal policy on human fetal research.

The bill also created a moratorium on federal support for fetal research until the report was completed (Capron 1989:22). According to one participant in the debates of this era, the possibility that the Department of Health Education and Welfare would act on the Ethics Advisory Board recommendation "still concerns many in Congress," which placed a new moratorium on the Secretary's granting any waivers for embryonic research (Capron 1989:23).

It took a year for Congress to appoint the Biomedical Ethics Board, and it took these directors two and a half years to appoint the members of the Commission that would actually do the work (Hanna, Cook-Deegan and Nishimi 1993:209). The directors from Congress were perfectly split over the abortion issue, and their fighting eventually meant that the budget for the group was cut off, and it died without ever doing anything (Bulger, Bobby and Fineberg 1995:94). Dueling social-movement organizations had effectively derailed public policy bioethics in this instance. Conservatives already had the ethical advice about fetal research that they needed, obtained from social-movement organizations in the religious right. Liberals already knew what they thought, too, receiving their ethical advice from the other side of the abortion debate.

In the late 1980s, the George H.W. Bush administration indefinitely extended an existing moratorium on federal funding of research on fetal tissue. Democrats introduced bills to override this ban, and one bill included a provision for the Ethics Advisory Board to review the research. This failed to pass. A bill passed in 1992, but was vetoed by President Bush, who in his veto message foregrounded his moral distaste for fetal tissue research (Hurlbut 2010:119). The antiabortion movement had continued to constrain public policy bioethics through elected officials.

Democrat William Clinton was elected president in 1992, and soon the NIH allowed funding of research on extra-corporeal human embryos. The NIH, back in Democratic hands, created a bioethics commission to address ethical issues having to do with embryos, creating the Human Embryo Research Panel (Hurlbut 2010:120).

Using the system of abstract knowledge of the bioethics profession, their method claimed to represent the reasonable ethical claims of all the citizens, not their own ethical views. The Panel concluded that it was ethical to conduct limited research on human embryos.

The chair of the commission reported that the majority of the speakers at the public presentation of the commission "represented an anti-abortion, 'pro-life' point of view. Roman Catholic religious publications and those of other anti-abortion organizations had alerted their readers to the panel's existence and had asked them to bring pressure to bear to prevent federal funding of embryo research" (Green 2001:59).

The method used by the bioethicists to create a microcosm of the public's ethics in their commission was not convincing to some conservative members of Congress. During the Panel's deliberations, a group of 35 senators—over a third of the Senate—wrote to the head of National Institutes of Health expressing concerns that the Panel would advocate the creation of embryos for their later destruction for research purposes. In a chapter of the chair's memoir titled "Politics Intrudes," which reflects the classical bioethical point of view that public policy bioethics exists to avoid politics, Ronald Green reported that the letter had text that "appeared to be borrowed from published articles by [the director of] the Catholic Secretariat for Pro-Life Activities, a sign that opponents of our work had friends in Congress" (Green 2001:91).

Toward the end of a series of long letters sent back and forth between the National Institutes of Health and the senators, the House of Representatives changed from Democratic to Republican control in the election symbolized by Newt Gingrich and the "Contract with America." In contrast to the five-page letters of earlier correspondence with Congress, after the election, the NIH received a five-sentence letter from famed antiabortion Republican House member Robert Dornan that simply said, "given the new realities of Congress . . . let it be known that we plan to use every legislative means available to prevent federal funds from being spent on grotesque research of this nature. I hope you will keep this in mind as you consider the recommendations of the Human Embryo Research Panel" (Hurlbut 2010:142). It was clear that the bioethics panel's work was unlikely to be accepted by religious conservatives, and that they were going to use their new political power to circumvent the public policy bioethics debate. They already had the ethical advice they needed on this issue, and it did not come from the public policy bioethics debate, but from social-movement organizations.

The White House, seemingly aware of the new conservative political environment, demanded that the head of NIH denounce the conclusions of his own Panel, but was rebuked. Only hours after the Panel publicly released its ethical recommendations, President Clinton counteracted the Panel and issued an executive order prohibiting the creation of embryos for research with federal money (Hurlbut 2010:141–42). Later it was reported that the decision was the result of "political forces that were bearing down on the White House" (Green 2001:104), not an alternative bioethical analysis. A year later, the Dickey-Wicker amendment was passed, which prohibits the use of Health and Human Services money for experiments that create, harm, or destroy embryos. The amendment was reportedly "high on the legislative agenda of the Christian Coalition, which had been stepping up pressure on Republicans to finally deliver results" (Green 2001:106). Dornan's threat had come true, and this amendment remained in force as of this writing (2009). Suffice it to say, antiabortion members of Congress do not accept the conclusions of bioethicists in public policy bioethics. Green concludes that government ethics commissions concerning reproduction "had repeatedly seen their work ignored or overturned by administration or congressional action," citing the fate of the 1979 Ethics Advisory Board report, the Fetal Tissue Transplantation Panel in the late 1980s, and his own 1995 embryo commission (Green 2001:105).

Finally, I turn to the Clinton-era bioethics commission, which used the method of common-morality principlism in the system of abstract knowledge of the bioethics profession to make its claims. They held a series of hearings about cloning in 1997, which included testimony from representatives of religious traditions. The publicly stated reasons for including religious voices were essentially that the public was very concerned about cloning, and since a majority of the public is religious, these voices must be included (Childress 1997; Evans 2002:190). Interviews of staff members of the Commission reveal that an additional reason why elite religious voices were included in the discussion after years of exile was "the concern that some congressional staff members expressed over the fact that there were no 'religious people' . . . on the Commission" (Messikomer, Fox and Swazey 2001:502). I think it is safe to say that the congressional representatives who pressured the Commission to include religious voices were being influenced by or were worried about the religious right, as there would be no other congressional constituency that would have wanted religious voices to be involved with the cloning debate.

While this group invited more religious people to testify than did previous commissions, the religious claims were transmuted into the language of principlism, thus seemingly transforming particular religious claims into universal American claims. Republicans were in the majority in the Senate, and Senator Bill Frist later organized a hearing titled "Ethical and Theological Implications of Cloning." Hurlbut's analysis is that, "for Frist this was an opportunity to advance a model of American pluralism that directly contradicted [National Bioethics Advisory Commission's]. He asserted that a problem like human cloning demands that the 'religious' be privileged in democratic discourse: 'theology must take its place in the public square'" (Hurlbut 2010:194). This is perhaps the antithesis of the bioethics profession's view, advocated by a prominent elected official, again suggesting that government officials were not accepting the methods of the bioethics profession.

The history of these commissions reveals that the jurisdiction-givers for public policy bioethics—elected and unelected government

officials—were increasingly ignoring bioethicists and instead turning to social movements for their ethical advice on beginning-and
end-of-life issues. However, the claim of the bioethics profession
that the social movements represented particular interests, while
bioethics was channeling the common morality, did not change,
despite prominent elected officials' not accepting it. The bioethics
profession soldiered on in a weakened state, perhaps saying that
issues having to do with embryos were too emotional to rationally
deal with. This strategy would fall apart with the election of
Republican George W. Bush.

Before the younger Bush, Ford was the last Republican president
who formed a general-issue government bioethics commission.
Carter created the commission that existed in the early Reagan era,
and the elder Bush did not have a commission. Then came the
Clinton years, followed by George W. Bush, who was certainly more
attentive to the concerns of the religious right than his father was.
While conservative social-movement activists were increasingly
giving ethical advice to government decision-makers, and apparently being listened to, it was the religious right's influence on
George W. Bush that would substantially damage the jurisdiction of
bioethics. Bush's bioethics commission would further challenge the
idea that the dominant methods of the bioethics profession produce
ethical recommendations based upon the public's values.

The President's Council on Bioethics

There is no topic more fraught for an analyst of bioethical debates
than Bush's commission, and I will try to bypass some of the emotional issues because they do not matter to the discussion at hand.
I will make the case that the members of the President's Council
used the system of abstract knowledge of the bioethics profession
and were, then, still bioethicists. But they rejected most of the
methods used by bioethicists. The distinct conclusions of these

bioethicists, compared to those of liberal bioethicists, and the reaction against their conclusions by liberal bioethicists, was the death knell for the legitimacy of the methods in the entire profession's system of abstract knowledge.

Modification of the Standard Methods in the System of Abstract Knowledge

This commission's methods were distinct from its predecessors'. Leon Kass was the first chair of the President's Council, and he clearly wanted to restructure the methods used in public policy bioethics that he thought had led to an impoverished debate in previous ethics commissions, and allow more room for diverse perspectives, including those from conservative religion. His central critique was that the methods of the bioethics profession had produced "thin" debates about pre-established ends, but not debates about what the ends of humanity should be:

> In brief, our first charge is a mandate to raise questions not only about the best means to certain agreed-upon ends, but also about the worthiness of the ends themselves, a mandate to be clear about all of the human goods at stake that we seek to promote or defend. It is a call to restore to public bioethics the concerns that gave rise to the field in the late 1960s and early 1970s: Where is biotechnology taking us? What does this mean for our humanity? . . . We are charged once again to thicken and enrich public bioethics discourse, away from the more limited, explicitly practical approaches adopted by the collaboration of scientists/physicians and professional bioethicists through the work of previous national commissions and regulatory bodies (Kass 2005:224–225).

This is an endorsement of condensed translation, and a rejection of transmutation of particularistic ends into preexisting ends to determine a common morality. That is, principlism was rejected outright as a method. Commissioners, Kass felt, should instead reflect upon what ends may be at stake and bring them to the group in a language that must be at least understood by the others. Typical of this focus on ends is the first paragraph in the first chapter of the Council's report titled *Beyond Therapy: Biotechnology and the Pursuit of Happiness*.

> What is biotechnology for? Why is it developed, used, and esteemed? Toward what ends is it taking us? To raise such questions will very likely strike the reader as strange, for the answers seem so obvious: to feed the hungry, to cure the sick, to relieve the suffering—in a word, to improve the lot of humankind, or, in the memorable words of Francis Bacon, "to relieve man's estate." Stated in such general terms, the obvious answers are of course correct. But they do not tell the whole story, and, when carefully considered, they give rise to some challenging questions, questions that compel us to ask in earnest not only, "What is biotechnology for?" but also, "What should it be for?" (President's Council on Bioethics 2003:1)

Kass was trying to bring bioethics back to the first or second era (see Chapter 1) of secular translations of ends. The concern with debating ends not only knocked common-morality principlism off the table as a method of generating the ethics of others, it also required rejecting the method of consensus among diverse commissioners. In the mandate for the Commission produced by the White House, directly formulated by Kass (Hurlbut 2010:200), it explicitly said the Commission would not strive for consensus, not wanting to paper over the value diversity that actually exists (Kass 2005:227–228). "There are only two ways to get consensus in such a public body," Kass would later write. "Either stack the council, losing all credibility, or seek agreement on the lowest common denominator issues—e.g., human cloning is 'at this time' unsafe—leaving all the big questions for some other body" (Kass 2005:227). He thought that consensus in the previous commissions had resulted in the vetoing of all but the thinnest of ethical conceptions.

The Challenge to the Consensus Among Diverse Commissioners Method

Principlism and consensus were creating the "thin" bioethical debate that Kass disliked, that ignored debates about ends. Yet, Kass was still by my definition a bioethicist, because he was trying to represent the values of the public in the ethical recommendations. The public would be represented by the commissioners, but his view of representativeness reflected the view that the method of having input from "diverse commissioners" used by bioethicists to that point resulted in commissioners who were not actually very representative.

Previous commissions in public policy bioethics had claimed to be representing the public through professional, gender, and racial diversity while avoiding the two types of diversity that actually matter to the public's views of bioethical issues—religious and educational diversity. First, consider "professional diversity." What this means in practice is that the commissions will have scientists and members of related professions like medicine, a social scientist or two, a lawyer or two, some philosophers and bioethicists, and a random academic from some other discipline. "Demographic diversity" means trying to include women and racial minorities. But why would we think that a social scientist would have different values from a physician? Why would we think that a woman has a different view from a man? Blacks and whites? Most studies that I am aware of about public attitudes toward the types of issues that bioethics deals with, such as beginning- and end-of-life issues, find two variables that produce the largest differences in opinion: education and religion. The differences between men and women and people of different races are either nonexistent or extremely small *on these sorts of issues.* (I have no doubt that if a commission debated affirmative action, the demographic variables would be relevant.)

The bottom line is that there is no diversity in values that matters on bioethics commissions that can solely be generated through demographic and professional diversity. All of those professionals were educated at the same modern research universities that make the same Enlightenment assumptions. Almost all hold a doctorate, a master's, or a doctor of law degree.[3] Similarly, religiously, commissioners either have not been identifiably religious or have been from a religious tradition that articulates with Enlightenment reasoning, such as mainline Protestantism, Reform or Conservative Judaism, or liberal Catholicism.

Religious conservatives probably concluded that this exclusion of conservative religious voices was intentional. A particularly egregious bias against members of certain religions on these commissions is exemplified by this exchange among the commissioners of the President's Commission of the early 1980s. Discussing a letter they received from mainline Protestant, Catholic, and Jewish leaders, and a newspaper article on the same subject, one commissioner remarked that:

> you will find that those churches—the Roman Catholic, the Episcopal, Presbyterian, Lutheran, and so forth—will have concerns quite similar to those that one might find in society in general. . . . That is not entirely true of certain other groups which use a religious language which has a more arcane meaning to that language. And the newspaper article we have here has reference to some of those groups, which might be called the fundamentalists. They will be included in a consensus, not just the ones who brought their concerns to us. So even in a religious area one has to make decisions about how people can be included in a more comfortable consensus.

While clearly this commissioner is trying to include fundamentalists, another commissioner breaks in to say "I don't know that [the executive director] has gotten such guidance" from the fundamentalists, to which another commissioner retorts, "He's not going to," resulting in laughter among the commissioners.[4] The lesson here is that only religious leaders who already agree with the general Enlightenment rationality of the other commissioners will be allowed a seat at the table. While this comment would never be made today because the jurisdiction-givers have changed, it is comments like this that have highlighted for conservatives that not all religious groups are represented on these commissions.

Moreover, in the method of consensus among diverse commissioners, there is explicitly to be no intentional ideological diversity. The Office of Technology Assessment report on public policy bioethics commissions claims that "[s]uccessful commissions were relatively free of political interference, had flexibility in addressing issues, were open in their process and dissemination of findings, and were comprised of a diverse group of individuals *who were generally free of ideology* and had wide ranging expertise."[5] Later, the report says that "[i]deology is a destructive criterion in appointing a bioethics committee. While selecting members solely on the basis of their stance on a particular issue—such as abortion—might be viewed by special interests as useful, such an approach is short sighted and likely to create gridlock" (U.S. Congress 1993:34).

Similarly, an Institute of Medicine study of bioethics commissions states that "in addition to 'the best that has been thought' on an issue, public ethics bodies should also be attentive to all the significant contributors to the public conversation about an issue" (Bulger, Bobby and Fineberg 1995:155). The reasons to be attentive to diverse contributions are: (a) these positions could be right; (b) if wrong, arguing against them strengthens the true case; (c) we should try to accommodate minority positions through policy; (d) failure to account for minority opinion may result in difficulty in policy implementation (Bulger, Bobby and Fineberg 1995:155–156). The representation of diverse views can come through membership on the commission, but, as they put it, "a seat at the table" should not be provided to people "who intend to champion a position and sway a deliberative body to accept it. This is undesirable for a public ethics body, which must be committed to impartiality and willingness to deliberate, yet the views of such parties deserve to be heard" (Bulger, Bobby and Fineberg 1995:156).

The most generous reading of these sorts of comments is that bioethicists think that commissions should avoid *ideologues*, those who come with fixed positions and have no intention of learning from each other. But, who are these people with doctorates in philosophy or medicine who have no ideology? For example, which philosopher is undecided about abortion? Does such a person exist? Who is the scientist who lacks a conclusion on whether the biomedical research enterprise should be encouraged or discouraged?

One person's blank slate is another person's ideologue. I suspect the conclusion of the religious right, operating through the Republican Party, was that, in practice, finding these "non-ideological" commissioners has meant adherence to the positions held by the mainstream of the bioethics profession and the profession of medicine and science. To take a couple of easy examples, name the last commissioner—before the George W. Bush commission—who was not a general enthusiast of medical and scientific research. Those who tend in this direction are not selected. Enthusiasm for medicine and science is not ideological, but "neutral," it appears. This is not a criticism of those who do serve on these commissions, some of whom I consider to be my friends. I know their positions are sincere—it is simply that their preexisting positions on these issues are among the reasons they were selected for this role. Technology critic Jeremy Rifkin, while articulating a somewhat widespread view in society, will never be on one of these commissions.

It is in this context that Kass's modification of the methods of the bioethics profession should be understood. Rejecting the bioethical method of finding professionally and racially diverse commissioners, he argued for finding ideologically diverse members. The method used by the President's Council for ensuring the common morality was diversity among commissioners in ideology and religion, without the consensus requirement.

Kass claimed to have a more diverse group of commissioners compared to previous commissions, writing that the Council was "the most intellectually diverse national bioethics council in recent history when it comes to embryo research—and, I would submit, also to most other things" (Kass 2005:226–227). He enumerated their professional diversity, and continued by writing that "by political leaning we are liberals and conservatives, Republicans, Democrats, and independents; and by religion we are Protestants, Catholics, Jews, and perhaps some who are none of the above" (Kass 2005:225–226).

The entire exchange between Kass and his critics about diversity of the commissioners and diversity in preset positions on embryos suggests that Kass believed that the views expressed in public policy bioethics contexts should mirror those of the general public (which is ideologically split on abortion and embryos.) Indeed, Kass claimed that Bush's Council was even *more* representative of the public's views than previous public policy bioethics commissions because "[l]ike the rest of the country, the President's Council on Bioethics is divided on ethics of embryo research. The same could not be said of the National Bioethics Advisory Council that served under President Clinton, a serious body that did some very valuable work, but a body without a single vote against embryo research—and no bioethicists, I believe, petitioned to complain" (Kass 2005:227). It is important to note that while claiming diversity, he was clearly focused upon religious or ideological diversity, not educational diversity, because this commission had the same or less educational diversity than previous commissions.[6]

Liberal Reaction and the Self-Delegitimization of the Bioethics Profession

Here was another government commission with the term *bioethics* in the title, claiming to represent the public's values even better than its predecessors—and it produced ethical recommendations quite at odds with those of the liberal wing of the profession. How the same "common morality" could lead to two ethical conclusions throws the entire profession into question. The reaction of the liberal wing of the bioethics profession to Bush's commission actually further revealed that the methods used previously by bioethicists do not result in representation of the common morality. The mainstream of the bioethics profession was spectacularly critical of this Council (Elliott 2004), with the primary complaint being that the Council actually was not diverse, but biased in a conservative direction. That is, the liberals denied that the conservatives are bioethicists by my definition, and said that they are not representing the general public's ethics in public policy bioethics. Liberals would say that while perhaps claiming this mantle, in actuality the members of the Bush Council were "stealth advocates" of particular normative, non-universal ethical positions (Briggle 2009).

For example, Arthur Caplan told an interviewer that one of the primary documents of the President's Council on Bioethics "was 'a politically conservative report' that espouses 'the quasi-religious view that the natural is good.'"[7] Kass himself summarizes the criticisms of the Council as being "a hyper-politicized group of right-wing Fundamentalists, seeking to impose pro-life views on the nation or to ignore scientific facts in the name of religious ideology" (Kass 2005:226). In an open letter to President Bush, signed by 170 bioethicists, many of whom headed the leading research centers in the field, the writers complained about the replacement of two Council members, writing that: "the creation of sound public policy with respect to developments in medicine and the life sciences requires a council that has a diverse set of views and positions.

By dismissing those two individuals and appointing new members whose views are likely to closely reflect those of the majority of the council and its chair the credibility of the council is severely compromised."[8] Liberal bioethicists' claims that the commissioners were not diverse simply demonstrated that this "diversity of commissioners" method was not going to lead to the public's accepting that the group represented the public's values.

The task in this task space is to recommend ethics to the government, and the bioethicists have jurisdiction based on their methods in their system of abstract knowledge that they claim produces ethics that represent the public's values, not their own, or the values of some particular group, like scientists. The earlier religious right challenges to government ethics commissions, and particularly the commission of George W. Bush, threw this into question. It will be hard for a future director of the National Institutes of Health to claim that the recommendations of an ethics commission are anything but the recommendations of a particular group of commissioners.

Where to Go From Here

We could end this story right here. The story would be called: "the end of the mirage of generating common morality on bioethical issues in the United States." Some critics have advocated exactly this (Engelhardt 2007). At present, the bioethics profession goes through the motions of creating commissions and other venues that purport to represent the common morality, but I think that nobody believes that the common morality is represented. The liberals did not recognize the Bush commission as representing the common morality, and the conservatives did not recognize the previous commissions as representing the common morality. Rather, each side has its affiliated social-movement organizations and its affiliated political party. What is depicted as the common morality now depends upon which particular group obtains political power.

As I will explain in Chapter 4, the emerging situation wherein social-movement activists give ethical advice *is* democratically legitimate. However, it is also a shame. Having different bioethical debates in the two political parties means that we do not learn from each other. Similarly, it is hard to imagine a fruitful discussion between the pro-choice and pro-life movement activists. Some on the extreme right will say that there is nothing to learn from the liberals, as their views are fundamentally corrupted. Those on the extreme left will say the same about the conservatives. For everybody else in the middle, the conversation would be useful.

The bioethics profession has three options in public policy bioethics. First, it can give up on representing the public, and each faction can be the ethical advisors to either the Democratic or Republican Party, depending upon who is in power. This is what I decry above. Second, bioethicists can hope that one side utterly destroys the other, so that the winner can say that they indeed represent the common morality with their methods and there is no legitimate voice to say otherwise. This seems extremely unlikely. Third, bioethicists can change the methods in their system of abstract knowledge so that it can withstand the charge that its methods do not result in the representation of the public's views. The methods for representing the people, such as common-morality principlism, can be modified to make them much more clearly represent the values of the public. This is what I advocate in the next section.

Notes

1. One possible exception would be Paul Ramsey, who, while a member of the mainline Protestant United Methodist Church, might today be considered a mainstream evangelical. For the counter-claim, see Hauerwas (1996).

2. (1) National Commission for the Protection of Human Subjects of Biomedical and Behavioral Research (1974–1978); (2) NIH Recombinant DNA Advisory Panel (1975–present); (3) Ethics Advisory Board

of the Department of Health, Education and Welfare (1978–1980); (4) President's Commission for the Study of Ethical Problems in Medicine and Biomedical and Behavioral Research (1980–1983); (5) Biomedical Ethics Advisory Committee (1988–1989); (6) Human Fetal Tissue Transplantation Research Panel, DHHS (1988); (7) Human Embryo Research Panel of the NIH (1994); (8) Advisory Committee on Human Radiation Experiments (1994–1995); (9) National Bioethics Advisory Committee (1996–2001); (10) President's Council on Bioethics (2001–2009); (11) Presidential Commission for the Study of Bioethical Issues (2009–).

3. For example, the National Bioethics Advisory Commission of the mid 1990s included seven Ph.D.s, three MDs, four J.D./LL.B.s, and four people who appear to not have had advanced degrees, but one of whom taught bioethics in a American research university. (See http:// bioethics.georgetown.edu/nbac/about/nbacroster.htm.) Similarly, the President's Commission of the early 1980s had six Ph.D.s (or equivalent), ten M.D.s, one J.D., one M.A. research scientist, and two people with bachelor's degrees (President's Commission 1983b). Moreover, if you look at the transcripts of meetings, the people without graduate degrees are less influential than the others.

4. President's Commission Meeting #11, p. 65, Kennedy Institute of Ethics Library.

5. My emphasis (U.S. Congress 1993:18).

6. For example, in the lists provided in the first and last reports of the Council, there are no commissioners who do not have advanced degrees. Some analysts claim that this is the result of Kass's Straussian philosophy that one should simply gather "persons considered the best thinkers" (Cohen 2005:283). I have yet to see any convincing evidence that the Council was influenced by Straussian thinking, however.

7. In Elliott (2004).

8. See http://bioethics.net/openletter.php (dated 3/25/2004).

PART III

Toward a New Era of
Bioethical Debate

Chapter 4

Task Clarification, Saying "No," and Making the Argument for Jurisdiction

Before suggesting reforms of the methods used by the bioethics profession that can solve the jurisdictional crisis in public policy bioethics, we have to clarify two issues. First, we must be much clearer about what the tasks in each of the jurisdictions actually are, and how the methods currently used by the bioethics profession make it more or less difficult to fulfill those tasks.

Second, we must also be more explicit than the bioethics profession ever has been about *why* it should be given jurisdiction over the task of recommending ethical policy that will be imposed upon all citizens of the country. Doctors are clear about why they should have jurisdiction over healing disease—they are better at it than faith healers. Bioethicists must be much more explicit in this regard. I will examine possible arguments for why bioethical conclusions should be structuring policy debates, and will conclude that the current claim to be representing the common morality *is* the best way to defend the profession's jurisdiction.

Watchdog Task

I have provided general descriptions of the tasks in the health-care ethics consultation and research bioethics task-spaces, but to see the origins of the crisis in the public policy bioethics jurisdiction we must be more specific. In addition to the task of mediating ethical disputes in health-care ethics consultation, and applying ethical regulations in the case of research bioethics, bioethicists have a task analogous to the watchdog's. The watchdog wanders around the property, not even doing anything, but the mere knowledge of the dog's presence precludes problems from happening. If anyone intrudes, it starts to bark and growl, probably stopping the intruder. If that does not stop the problem, it can then bite. Critically, the watchdog does not create the rules but is enforcing the rules of the master, such as "no nocturnal theft." Analogously, in professional jurisdiction terms, a profession with a watchdog task cannot create its methods or system of abstract knowledge on its own.

In research bioethics, the task is to be the watchdog by enforcing the established system of ethics set by the federal government, not to create one's own ethical system. In health-care ethics consultation, mediating ethical disagreements is not a watchdog task, but the task of making sure that these ethical decisions stay "within the bounds of ethical and legal standards" is such a task (American Society for Bioethics and Humanities 2011:10). The American Society for Bioethics and the Humanities core competency report for ethics consultation recommends that the dog not growl often, but be prepared to. They write that "although the ethics consultation service should never function as 'the ethics police,' the consultant should notify the involved parties that, like others, they may be obligated to report egregious violations to supervisors or oversight bodies." *Egregious violation* includes "obvious violations of law, hospital policy, professional codes of ethics or an organizational code of conduct or ethical norm" (American Society for Bioethics and Humanities 2011:8). Bioethicists are then the watchdogs for externally derived "codes of ethics" and "ethical norms." Most critically, in both research bioethics and health-care ethics consultation, the watchdog must be inside the house to see any possible violations in process. But who is the master who owns the house and creates the rules?

Jurisdictional Settlements

To understand being the watchdog inside the house as the task, I must import one last idea from the sociology of professions—settlements in the jurisdictional space. Professions generally compete for full jurisdiction over particular work. Medicine is the classic case of full jurisdiction, where those not in the profession who engage in tasks that the profession has jurisdiction over (like surgery) are put in jail. Some professions—perhaps seeing their limited chances for obtaining full jurisdiction in competition with a strong incumbent—reach settlements with each other regarding where the boundaries between two professions will lie. Bioethics has never had full jurisdiction in any of its jurisdictions, but has always had less powerful jurisdictions.

The bioethics profession has a settlement with the medical/scientific professions that Abbott calls "subordination," where a dominant profession gives subsidiary acts to another.[1] The classic cases of subordination include doctors and nurses, or doctors and X-ray technicians. Nurses and X-ray technicians do not have their own system of abstract knowledge, but rather use that of their superior profession, and the superior profession defines the tasks. Analogously, the tasks in the health-care ethics consultation and public policy bioethics were originally defined by the medical/scientific professions, and the actual principles in the common-morality principlist method in the system of abstract knowledge of the bioethics profession are based on the values of the medical/scientific professions. The bioethics profession is then the watchdog for the medical/scientific professions' ethics in the health-care ethics consultation and research bioethics task-spaces.

Note again that this sociological understanding of professions does not presume that there was the professional equivalent of a Yalta Conference where leaders signed a treaty that would divide the available task-space. Rather, equivalent arrangements evolved as individual actors reacted to social pressures. In this case, individual bioethicists who wrote or spoke in a way that assumed too much "territory" were discouraged, and those who wrote or spoke in a way that assumed the settlement were encouraged. For example, the legislation creating the second federal government bioethics commission required that three commissioners be from biomedical and behavioral research and three from medicine (Evans 2002:253). If a bioethicist had suggested to the member of Congress drafting this legislation that no scientists be allowed on the commission because bioethicists should have full jurisdiction, they would have been ignored because the scientific community would have protested their exclusion.

The Subordinate Jurisdiction of the Bioethics Profession

The claim of subordinate jurisdiction is in contrast to the common self-image of the bioethics profession as an oppositional movement to science and medicine. While the bioethics profession did take over tasks from science/medicine while defeating the theologians, they took over in a way that did not harm medicine/science. The professions have never been in serious competition. I concur with historian Charles Rosenberg that

> bioethics not only questioned authority; it has in the past quarter-century helped constitute and legitimate it. As a condition of its acceptance, bioethics has taken up residence in the belly of the medical whale; although thinking of itself as still autonomous, the bioethical enterprise has developed a complex and symbiotic relationship with this host organism. Bioethics is no longer (if it ever was) a free-floating, oppositional, and socially critical reform movement (Rosenberg 1999:37–38).

To understand this claim, we should start with the fact that the tasks in these two task-spaces were created by scientists and physicians before the theologians or the bioethicists entered these debates. A profession that gets to initially define the task is going to define it in such a way that it supports their other jurisdictions. Health-care ethics consultation had existed for centuries—it was just so totally under the jurisdiction of doctors that it was not considered to be separate from their other jurisdictions. The task of health-care ethics consultation as originally designed fits with doctors' other jurisdictions, such as treating disease in hospitals— in fact, the task is intentionally narrow so that it fits with the other tasks. Similarly, the task in research bioethics was originally "part of" being a good research scientist, and was limited to the sorts of tasks that would support research. The new task-space would not fundamentally challenge the other jurisdictions of the profession. One of the reasons that contemporary research bioethics cannot be used to challenge the jurisdictions of the research scientists—by, for example, asking whether it is always good to have more scientific knowledge—is that research scientists originally designed the task-space to be supportive of their other jurisdictions.

When bioethicists gained their subsidiary jurisdiction over these tasks, they did not challenge the boundaries of the tasks as they had been defined by doctors and scientists. For example, in health-care ethics consultation, bioethicists still considered the task to be one of resolving the *individual* medical dilemma involving an *individual* patient, not larger debates about, for example, whether hospitals should be profit-making. Similarly, in research bioethics, scientists had already defined the task in similarly individualistic terms—"should this one particular experiment (not a class of experiment) go forward?" and the only relevant issue was the effects on research subjects, not the effect on society, or questions about the purpose of science.

It is not only that science/medicine defined these two task-spaces, but that the methods originally used for making ethics decisions by science/medicine structured the subsequent methods developed by bioethicists. For example, the current principles used by the bioethics profession were largely derived by observing the "best practices" of scientists, so principlism is closely related to a method that scientists and physicians could have come up with on their own. The National Commission—which first articulated the principles—conducted a number of investigations of the treatment of human research subjects, examining whether, for example, subjects had actually given their informed consent, or whether the risk was actually as minimal as was claimed by the researchers. The nascent bioethics profession *did* innovate in creating the principle of "respect for persons" to justify the by-then long-standing practice of informed consent, but if one starts with the practice of informed consent, there is only a limited range of principles that can be created. Similarly, "beneficence"—doing good and avoiding harm—has always been central to medicine, as embodied in strictures like "first, do no harm," traditionally attributed to the Hippocratic Oath. The conflict between science and the nascent bioethics profession was not over the content of the principles, but rather that scientists and doctors—like all professionals— wanted to use their own discretion in applying these principles. My conclusion about the early days of the nascent bioethics profession is that bioethicists forced the scientists and physicians to clarify and rigorously apply the procedures that had supposedly already been put in place by the scientists. The principles behind the procedures were not controversial.

One exception was the procedure of selecting research subjects, and many of the scandals that emerged in the 1960s and 1970s involved research on people seemingly selected because they lacked social power, like orphans, prisoners, and poor African-American men. The Belmont Report emphasized a somewhat new principle of "justice" to the selection of research subjects. For example, researchers could not use orphans for research solely for the reason that orphans were readily available. Even if you think it was the "chicken" of the values pushed by the bioethics profession instead of the "egg" of medical/scientific values, they are now the same. The bioethics profession's task is to enforce the internal values of the medical/scientific profession *in these two task-spaces*.

The subordinate role of the bioethics profession in the two jurisdictions is also indicated by the fact that in the first organizational moments of bioethical debate in the late 1960s and early 1970s, before the emergence of the bioethics profession, the first research centers were independent of the medical and scientific enterprise. The Hastings Center, arguably the first bioethics center, was free-standing, unrelated to any university or medical school. The Kennedy Institute of Ethics at Georgetown University, founded in the same era, was more associated with the philosophy and theology departments than with the medical school (Jonsen 1998:22–24). Now, with a profession of bioethics with subordinate jurisdiction over research bioethics and health-care ethics consultation, bioethics centers are largely part of medical schools and often dependant on them for their funding.[2] Moreover, these centers are largely dependent on grant income, and the granting entities, such as the NIH, are controlled by scientists, so scientists get to define the important questions.

The medicine/science profession originally did not want to share jurisdiction, and originally the bioethics profession probably wanted a stronger jurisdiction. However, it was a forced marriage of sorts, with the shotgun being held by the federal government, which clearly was not going to entirely override the desires of scientists. For example, critical policies in the development of the jurisdiction were put in place by the precursors to the NIH, which is closely aligned with the science profession.

The settlement was beneficial to the physicians and scientists because, at the time, their ethics were distrusted, due to the scandals on their watch. What the bioethics profession brought to the arrangement was a profession that was *not* the distrusted medical/scientific profession, and, more important, the claim that it would ensure that the new values used in the medical/scientific profession were actually based upon the values of the citizens.

If the arguments of bioethicists ever strayed far from the interests of the medical/scientific profession, the medical/scientific profession would have already tried to kill off bioethics. With many prominent bioethics centers embedded in medical schools, dependent on their legitimacy and largess, it seems unlikely that if the bioethics and the medical/scientific professions were really competitors, one competitor would allow the other to live in its house. In sum, they are not competitors, but have a settlement *in these two task-spaces*. The ethics of the bioethics profession is the same as the ethics of science and medicine, and the bioethicists' task is to enforce these ethics in the houses of scientific research and health-care practice.

The Problems With the Subordinate Jurisdictions

Of course the problem with having subordinate jurisdiction is that you cannot question the system of abstract knowledge held by the superior profession, and that is one reason professions strive for full jurisdiction. For example, nurses cannot change surgical techniques, even though they participate in surgeries. For an insider, critique also becomes difficult or impossible. Watchdogs that growl at their owners will be replaced. Albert Dzur concludes that "rather than being a strong voice of critique, bioethics developed as a form of 'regulatory ethics,' something that allowed ethicists a more powerful internal role in organized medicine" (Dzur 2008:212). Sociologist Charles Bosk concurs, describing bioethics as "a contemporaneous alternative to a more forceful challenge to medicine spearheaded by consumer and patient activists. This later challenge was more confrontational in tone, more insistent on structural change, and more focused on the politics of health care than was the bioethics movement. By assimilating bioethics, organized medicine was able to defang this other, broader challenge" (Bosk 1999:64).

Dzur sums this perspective up quite nicely using a political science term, the *institutional capture* of bioethics by science and medicine. Linking the idea of institutional capture to the inability of bioethics to raise issues that are contrary to the interests of the science/medicine profession, Bosk continues that a captured bioethics has "not raised a number of political issues that also can be defined as ethical questions: the presence of so many millions of Americans without health insurance, the multiple ways the production pressures of managed care undercut the possibilities of the doctor–patient relationship that bioethics celebrates, the inequalities in health status between rich and poor, or the replacement of professional values with corporate ones" (Bosk 1999:64).

The Advantages of the Subordinate Jurisdictions

The subordinate jurisdictional task of being the watchdog for the tasks defined by the medical/scientific profession, and using their ethics, has ultimately been positive for the bioethics profession and for ethical behavior more generally. The watchdog role has simply meant that criticism of the medical/scientific system of ethics enforced by the bioethics profession or criticism of medicine and science generally cannot come from the bioethics profession itself, but from outside, which has largely been the case (as in the book you are currently reading). However, given what bioethicists saw as the ethical problems at the time this settlement evolved, the insider watchdog task probably allowed them to be the most effective at ending ethical abuses. For example, while there have been ethical lapses by medical researchers, there has been nothing that has reached the level of a Tuskegee scandal since the imposition of IRBs.[3] This is quite an accomplishment. By being literally inside of the hospitals with health-care ethics consultation and inside the scientific research enterprise with IRBs, bioethics is in a position to actually prevent ethics abuses from happening. You have to be inside the fence to guard the house. The task could not be conducted by a profession that was *not* allowed to be on the inside.

An insider position is useful for a second reason, which is that, by behaving like insiders instead of outsider revolutionaries, bioethicists who give suggestions to people in science and medicine with actual power (like the dean of a medical school or hospital administrator) may find that these are actually followed instead of resisted. Overall, I think the jurisdictional settlement between bioethics and science/medicine in these two task-spaces is effective, and I do not advocate that it be changed.

Subordinate Jurisdiction in Public Policy Bioethics Harms the Bioethics Profession

The bioethics profession also has a subordinate jurisdiction in public policy bioethics. Again, there were people at the founding of the task-space and the initial awarding of jurisdiction who wanted jurisdiction to be more independent of the science/medicine profession, including senators Mondale and Kennedy. The influence of the scientists was too strong, and what was available was the subordinate jurisdiction eventually taken by the bioethics profession.

While the tasks in research bioethics and health-care ethics consultation can only be conducted if the profession is allowed to be inside (i.e., in a subordinate relationship to science/medicine), the subordinate role vis-à-vis science/medicine in public policy bioethics has been damaging the ability of bioethicists to hold jurisdiction from nearly the beginning. The reason is that the task in public policy bioethics itself—which was not invented by scientists—requires being able to say "no" to scientists, and the subordinate arrangement makes that difficult.

The Bioethics Profession in Public Policy Bioethics Rarely Says "No"

Many observers have noted that while the bioethics profession regularly says "no" to scientists in the research bioethics task-space, and says "no" to doctors in the health-care ethics consultation task-space, it rarely says "no" in public policy bioethics. For example, Daniel Callahan writes that

> while bioethics creates problems now and then for main-stream, right-thinking trends, it mainly serves to legitimate them, adding the imprimatur of ethical expertise to what somebody or other wants to do. It is hardly likely that the National Institutes of Health (NIH) Human Genome Project would have set aside 5 percent of its annual budget for the Ethical, Legal, and Social Implications program if there had been even the faintest likelihood it would turn into a source of trouble and opposition; and it indeed hasn't (Callahan 1996:3).[4]

Political scientist Langdon Winner, in congressional testimony, gives the strong version of this critique, saying that: "the professional field of bioethics has a great deal to say about many fascinating things, but people in this profession rarely say 'no.' . . . Indeed, there is a tendency for career-conscious social scientist and humanists to become a little too cozy with researchers in science and engineering, telling them exactly what they want to hear" (*Nature* editorial 2006). Even more strongly, Leon Kass argues that bioethics must be "more than an exchange of sanctimonious permission slips for unrestrained scientific freedom and technological innovation" (Kass 2005:246).

Retaining Jurisdiction in Public Policy Bioethics Requires the Possibility of Saying "No"

While the jurisdiction-giver is the government official, the government official must be aware of what elected officials think, and elected officials in turn must be aware of what the public thinks. As noted in the last chapter, the public, through social movements, has increasingly paid attention to these issues. The possibility of saying "no" is required because the public does not want scientists to have carte blanche in developing new technologies. For example, the 2006 General Social Survey asked respondents, "When making policy recommendations about stem-cell research," to what extent do you think scientists "would support what is best for the country as a whole versus what serves their own narrow interests?" While scientists were considered to be the least self-interested group asked about (the others being elected officials and business leaders), on a scale of one to five, 34% of respondents selected "one," which is that scientists will do what is best for the country. 27% selected "two," and the remaining 39% leaned more toward the view that scientists will advance "their own narrow interests." The same question asked about global warming found 42% selecting the "what is best for the country" end of the scale, 28% the next more-critical response, and the remainder were more toward the response that scientists are advancing their own narrow interests. While the scientific community is not deeply distrusted like elected officials, I think it is safe to say that the public is unsure whether the scientific community is acting in the public interest.

If these questions had asked about whether we should follow the *ethics* of scientists, I think the numbers would show even less deference. So, while a goodly sized section of the public trusts scientists to be acting in the public interest, another large segment of the public disagrees. Importantly for the case I made in the last chapter, those who do not want to trust scientists are disproportionately conservative Protestants. For example, among members of conservative Protestant denominations who attend services regularly, 33% think climate scientists operate in the public interest, compared to the 43% of non-conservative Protestants who feel this way. Similar findings can be found in the question about embryonic stem-cell research (Davis, Smith and Marsden 2008).[5]

If the public does not think that scientists should be able to engage in any technology they develop, and the task in the public policy bioethics task-space is to debate this very question, if the bioethics profession can only say "yes" to scientists, then it will have no credibility; and to the extent government officials are responsive to the public, bioethicists will lose jurisdiction. Among people who trust scientists even less (e.g., conservative Protestants) bioethics will have even less credibility, and if government officials start listening to conservative Protestants, bioethics will have an even more threatened jurisdiction. This is of course what has been happening. To retain jurisdiction, a reformed bioethics profession needs to be able to say "no" in public policy bioethics.

Determinants of the Inability to Say "No"

Perhaps the bioethics profession's jurisdiction over public policy bioethics was destined to be unstable from the beginning. It is the definition of the task and the content of principlism, that leads to not being able to say "no" in *public policy bioethics*. This is not due to some conspiracy whereby bioethicists receive memos with instructions from the National Institutes of Health or are secretly trying to allow scientists to do as they wish. It is much subtler, as even an "anti-science" bioethicist would end up saying 'yes."

The first reason why bioethicists seem to be unable to say "no" in public policy bioethics is the flow of issues between the task-spaces. When a new controversial scientific development appears, such as synthetic biology, discussion of it starts in cultural bioethics. It inevitably starts with a newspaper article that reports that some scientist or physician would like to engage in new technology X. To take a few examples, reproductive cloning needed to be debated because some scientist may decide to try to do it; synthetic biology was being conducted by private labs; germline human genetic engineering was increasingly seen by scientists as a way to effectively control disease; and a clinic in California wanted to start screening embryos for skin color. This is debated in the public sphere through the media.

If there is a faction of the participants in the cultural bio-ethics debate who have political influence and question whether the scientific or medical innovation should be done, the issue then moves to the public policy bioethics task space. For example, creating stem cells from adult skin cells is a discussion in cultural bioethics, but there is nobody who thinks this should stop, so it has not entered public policy bioethics. On the other hand, discussion of embryonic stem-cell research entered cultural bioethics when this technique was discovered. It soon traveled to public policy bioethics as a group of people wanted this research to stop. Should policy be created to encourage or discourage scientists from doing this?

If bioethicists in public policy bioethics successfully describe the ethics of the new technology in the language of principlism, then any ethical issues about the new technology can by definition be handled by ethical analysis in the research bioethics task-space. The ethical problem has been redefined from one to be discussed in the public policy bioethics jurisdiction with unknown and controversial ethical implications, to one with well understood and ordinary ethical dilemmas that should be discussed in research bioethics. If it is in research bioethics, it is an issue that research can begin on, because the task is to evaluate *proposed* research studies where the ethical problems can be handled routinely. A successful transmutation to principlism in public policy bioethics always means "yes," because transmutation makes the issue a research bioethics issue.

For example, when it was decided that somatic cell human gene therapy could be described in the public policy bioethics jurisdiction using principlism, it then became part of acceptable medical research, and thus was under the jurisdiction of bioethicists in the research bioethics task-space (Evans 2002:Ch. 4). Therefore, since principlism is used in public policy bioethics to transmute claims into the ethical system also used in research bioethics, it does not say "no" to new technologies. This in turn damages the jurisdictional claim of bioethicists, because a profession is not really fulfilling the task of evaluating and recommending ethical public policy on scientific and medical issues if its own system of evaluation always results in a "yes." "No" in public policy bioethics comes from claims that resist transmutation.

A second reason bioethicists tend to not say "no" is that the current principles used in public policy bioethics were invented by physicians and scientists for *individual* decision-making in research trials and health-care decisions. The principles are then not capable of addressing the *social* decision-making required in public policy bioethics. When social decisions are transmuted into an individualist ethical decision-making system, it tends to be up to any individuals affected by a technology to decide what to do (e.g., say "yes"). Many readers will recognize this as part of what Adam Hedgecoe calls the "social science critique" of the bioethics profession's system of abstract knowledge: that for bioethicists, "the individual is the proper measure of all things ethical" (Hedgecoe 2004:125).[6] For example, "autonomy" asks in research bioethics and health-care ethics consultation whether Jane Smith, the research subject or patient, has given her informed consent to be experimented upon or be treated. For non-maleficence, the question is: Will one of the 100 people who ingest this drug be harmed by it (research bioethics), or, Will brain surgery on Patient X be too risky? (heath-care ethics consultation). "Autonomy" on a social level is almost nonsensical. "Justice" is potentially a social concept, but is not really used much by bioethicists outside of research bioethics (Jonsen 1998:413).

While "harm" works well in the individually oriented tasks in research bioethics and health-care ethics consultation because it is equated with something considered to be objective (physical damage to the body), "harm" to society is much more elusive and non-consensual. For example, non-bioethicists who compete with bioethicists for jurisdiction in cultural bioethics often raise the issue of cultural harms, such as the idea that certain technologies will harm humanity's conception of itself. Cultural harms cannot be effectively described using an individualistic ethical system like principlism, so if these concerns cannot be transmuted into principlism, they are discarded, effectively discarding much of the criticism of a technology. This results in an inability to say "no" to an emergent technology using principlism.

Consider somatic human genetic engineering, wherein the genes of a person are changed to try to heal a disease. (*Germline* engineering would change the genes of the person and all of their descendants'.) There were many socially stated concerns about this technology. Somatic engineering was originally controversial, and considered outside of the bounds of medicine. Then bioethicists and scientists successfully made the case that such treatments fit within a principlist ethical framework, and somatic engineering became ethical and a legitimate part of medical research (Evans 2002). Subsequently, scientists said that they were close enough to being able to engage in *germline* human genetic engineering that an ethical debate should begin, to see if it, too, could be described by principlism and therefore become acceptable experimental practice under the research bioethics jurisdiction. In this debate, scientists and bioethicists tended to argue that germline human genetic engineering fit with principlism—it forwarded beneficence, nonmaleficence, autonomy, and justice. This type of analysis revealed that it was ethical and, by extension and following bioethics' relationship with science/medicine, germline human genetic engineering should be part of medical research (Evans 2002).

When constrained to the use of principlism, social concerns such as "what should be the purpose of human evolution?" had to be transmuted into one of the individually expressed principles. The only way to argue for intergenerational purpose using the current principles is to ask whether the autonomous decision-making of people who do not yet exist would be violated, as they have not given their permission to be experimented upon (Evans 2002). Surely, if one were opposed to germline human genetic engineering, and not constrained to using the current principles, one would come up with a better argument than this. Once it is safe, I predict that germline human genetic engineering will become part of the tasks of the medical profession, because there is no way to make social arguments against it using the current version of individualist principlism.

Finally, the other primary method of the bioethics profession—consensus among diverse commissioners—also tends to not say "no." This is because scientists are always one of the "diverse professions" in government ethics commissions, and typically the group with the largest representation. This fact itself is evidence of bioethics' subordinate relationship to science/medicine. Would the American Medical Association allow chiropractors onto its panel deciding best practices for back pain? Would a modern-day council of Nicaea allow non-theologian competitors—say Richard Dawkins—to help determine the nature of the Trinity? That is not what a profession with full jurisdiction does. If the bioethics profession really had full jurisdiction over the ethics of science, there would not be scientists on government bioethics commissions. Of course, non-scientists need to have the scientific issues explained to them, but scientists could be brought in as consultants for that task. Why are they commissioners? It was clear from the founding of the first government ethics commission that scientists would have strenuously protested any commission that did not give scientists a strong voice (Jonsen 1998:90–98).

The consensus among diverse commissioners method requires that any ethical conclusion be consistent with the scientists' ethics. How does this veto power work? Imagine you are a professor, and when your department tries to hire a new professor, the procedure in the committee is to have each member go through all of the files and come back with 10 candidates that they want to discuss further in committee, so that a shorter list of candidates to discuss can be made. Except one of the members of the committee comes back with only one candidate and says "none of the rest are acceptable to me." "Consensus" in this procedure means that this one faculty member dictatorially selects future professors.

Something similar is inevitable when consensus involves a group that has a very constrained version of ethics (analogous to liking only one job candidate). In my analyses of commissions, I have found that it is the bench scientist and ordinary M.D. commissioners who have a very constrained version of ethics. (This is not the case for the much rarer polymath scientist or physician.) The ordinary scientist or physician commissioner believes very strongly in relieving human suffering. Indeed, that is probably why they became scientists and physicians, and many see suffering on a daily basis, so they want to see technologies that can relieve suffering proceed. They are also very interested in discoveries about nature. Obviously these are noble goals and are shared by the other commission members. However, their ethical concerns tend to stop there, whereas the other commissioners bring a wider range of ethical concerns to the table. Of course, some scientists may have additional values and concerns, but they did not derive them from their day jobs, as I would argue that the institution of science in the United States—particularly at the elite level—only teaches the relief of suffering and the value of discovery as important values. Like the colleague who only selects one job candidate to discuss, the only consensus one can reach with a commissioner like this is that the ethical value of relieving suffering and making discoveries about nature should be maximized. This means in practice that ethical concerns about a technology that cannot be transmuted to beneficence and non-maleficence will not achieve consensus as legitimate concerns, and the consensus method means that principlism needs to be used, with all the attendant problems described above. In sum, these forces that lead to not being able to say "no" in public policy bioethics need to be accounted for in the reforms I suggest in the next chapter.

Toward Creating a Clear Justification for Jurisdiction

One impediment to retaining jurisdiction in public policy bioethics is that bioethicists have not clearly stated why they should be given jurisdiction, perhaps due to a lack of reflection on the topic. Doctors are quite clear why they should have jurisdiction over healing disease—they are better at it than acupuncturists; and bioethicists should develop a similar level of clarity.

The tasks in the three jurisdictions are very particular, and all involve making ethical recommendations for policies that are *binding on all of the citizens*. For example, if the government pays for embryonic stem-cell research, we all pay for this research. If you try to assert that you are going to pay less in taxes because you do not support embryonic stem-cell research, you will be put in jail. Similarly, a hospital is not going to create a personalized health-care ethics consultation method for you, but rather you will have to take what they offer everyone.

The justification for the bioethicists' jurisdiction in public policy bioethics has been particularly vague, and it is here I will focus my energy. I agree with Gary Belkin, who claims that "bioethicists have not generally included in their work questions such as 'How is it that I am in a position to address these particular kinds of questions in the forms and approaches I do, and to the audience and with the authority and sponsor I have?'" (Belkin 2004:378). Therefore, in creating a defensible method for this particular task-space we must pay attention to what is going to be accepted by the public as a reason for why bioethicists can give advice to the government on a policy issue.

Anyone giving advice to the government needs to have a reason that they can legitimately do so. Of course, any citizen can legitimately give advice to the government by writing a letter to their elected official. However, bioethicists do not claim to be speaking as average citizens, for if they were, they would not accept opportunities that allow them a more direct channel to elected officials, such as being a member of a government ethics commission or publishing an article recommending a policy for the NIH. Ordinary citizens cannot legitimately claim either of those ways of giving advice. Let us go through some possible justifications for giving advice to policy-makers that I could use in recommending reforms of the bioethics profession.

Interest-Group Liberalism

To make a more powerful claim than what one is allowed as an ordinary citizen, you have to legitimately claim to be representing something larger than yourself. How is this done? One form of political legitimacy is interest-group liberalism, where democracy is based upon the actions of interest groups and social movements—like the American Medical Association, the National Organization for Women, and the Christian Coalition—who represent groups of like-minded citizens in the public sphere. These groups pressure the government to forward the interests of their members (Pateman 1970).

Of course, bioethicists could transform themselves into social movement activists and theoretically retain legitimacy, becoming the house intellectuals for the social movements described in Chapter 3 such as the right-to-life movement, the pro-choice movement, and the Catholic Church. If a former bioethicist in this context were to suggest that the NIH not fund embryonic stem-cell research, the person would have legitimacy because they are the representative of the citizens who are members of the organization, each of whom has a right to advise the government.

The interest-group model is also at work if bioethicists base their legitimacy on representing an elected official, such as the president (Johnson 2006). The suggested ethical policies would be democratically legitimate because they are an extension of the president's legitimacy, and ethical suggestions would be expected to fit with the president's agenda. If the religious right, working through the Republican Party, elects their candidate as president, the ethics of the liberals will not be represented.

Interest-group legitimation is where these government ethics commissions are headed, with President Bush's President's Council on Bioethics being portrayed as serving only the Republican Party's ethics, and President Obama disbanding Bush's Council before its time was even done. Public policy bioethics more broadly is also becoming more like dueling interest groups. For example, liberals have set up "progressive bioethics" associated with organs of the Democratic Party (Moreno and Berger 2010). While democratically legitimate, an interest group legitimation for the bioethics profession would lead to the end of public policy bioethics as we know it, and lead to two distinct public policy bioethics debates: a Democratic one and a Republican one, with the group out of power forming a sort of shadow debate. Obviously bioethics could no longer claim to not be representing a subgroup of the population. Developing this type of legitimacy is not a solution to the jurisdictional crisis; it will deepen the jurisdictional crisis.

Representing the Common Morality

Methods like principlism and consensus among diverse commissioners claim an expansion of the logic of interest-group liberalism. Whereas in interest-group liberalism people speak for the interests of some segment of the population, common-morality theories claim legitimacy because they are speaking for the interests of the entire population.

I would argue that one of the reasons for the degree of success of the bioethics profession is that it has at least quietly claimed this legitimation device. When bioethicists make ethical claims about controversial issues such as stem-cell research, the underlying claim of common morality gives them the additional legitimacy that justifies a bioethicist's being given an audience: they are representing the entire public's actual views. The claim of a common morality means that bioethicists are implicitly more legitimate than representatives of interest groups, because interest groups are by definition not representing *all* of the citizens, but only an interested faction. For example, it is easy to argue that the Christian Coalition does not represent the views of the entire public.

Technocratic Legitimation

To the extent the bioethics profession is explicit in its claims for jurisdiction in public policy bioethics, it claims to be legitimate because it represents the common morality. However, the actual operation of its methods gives the appearance that the profession claims a different form of legitimacy for making public policy recommendations—technocratic legitimation. This, then, is one of the primary defects in the bioethicists' methods that will need to be repaired.

Technocratic legitimation speaks for "facts" or "truth"—"a system of governance in which technically trained experts rule by virtue of their specialized knowledge and position in dominant and political and economic institutions" (Fischer 1990:17). This notion goes back to Plato's call for philosopher kings, and Francis Bacon's idea that technical elites should rule to maximize efficiency and technical order (Fischer 1990:67). It is not simply that the average layperson cannot give advice on whether a river provides enough water to cool a nuclear power plant—and that experts are needed for this task—but that in a technocracy, technical solutions are offered for problems that were at one time considered to be political problems of conflicting values and interests. Technocracy removes the values of the public from consideration. In one theorist's description:

> To ask a politician, let alone the person on the street, to make decisions about complex issues like nuclear power is said to be archaic. Neither the politician nor the everyday citizen has the information and sophistication to deal with such decisions. Albeit unpalatable to many, the technocratic solution is seen to be foreordained: political issues must be redefined in scientific or technical terms. This is the job of experts. They must be brought to the fore (Fischer 1990:22–23).

Therefore, the first characteristic of technocracy for our purposes is a "deep-seated animosity toward politics itself" and toward the public's ability to make decisions (Fischer 1990:16). But, it is not just that with technocracy, experts will rule. The second, and more important characteristic of technocracy is that expert rule is justified by making policy decisions *seem to be* only about facts, which are fixed; not values, which vary from group to group. This is accomplished by removing debates about values in politics and making political decisions solely about selecting the most efficacious means for forwarding taken-for-granted values. Centeno, studying Mexican politics, recognized the "rule of experts" as one component of technocracy, but considered this removal of debates over values to be perhaps an even more important characteristic of technocracy (Centeno 1997:314).

As an example, a debate about the Mexican economy is technocratic if it is considered to be a fact that economic efficiency is the preeminent value, and the debate is to determine which means will then maximize economic efficiency. A debate about the Mexican economy would not be technocratic if there were first or concurrently a debate over what values to pursue through economic policy, and then a debate on the means to use to achieve the decided values. Technocratic debates do not only occur in Mexico. For example, education policy debates assume the fact that the United States needs to have "the highest level of intellectual achievement for children," although upon occasion people try to reopen debate by asking, for example, what "achievement" is.

Other scholars have noted a technocratic impulse in the bioethics profession, where information about the values of the public is actually not considered. In their review of the democratic legitimation of bioethics commissions, Dzur and Levin see the temptation to technocracy among bioethicists as strong enough that they spend a substantial number of words arguing against it (Dzur and Levin 2004). Similarly, Mark G. Kuczewski writes that "bioethics commissions should not allow the values of their members to lead them to delegitimize the values of sizable portions of the citizenry. That is, as professional academics, bioethicists may be more inclined to value the advancement of science than the average person and to value sanctity of life considerations less than much of the general public" (Kuczewski 2007:92).

Howard Brody also describes a technocratic impulse in the bioethics profession that grows as one moves from health-care ethics consultation to public policy bioethics, with an imaginary story:

> Mr. Smith lies in the intensive care unit. There is a dispute about whether he should be maintained on a ventilator, or started on renal dialysis. . . .
>
> Our initial response to the consultation request will be both unanimous and vociferous. Let Mr. Smith speak for himself. We must hear the voice of the patient—the voice that for too many decades or centuries, the paternalistic practice of medicine sought to ignore or suppress. . . .
>
> But now, let Mr. Smith arise from his bed. Let him put on his clothes and walk out of the hospital. Let him go about his daily business in the community. Suddenly, our bioethicists' insistence that his voice be heard dissipates. In our bioethics work, we read what each other has written; we teach our classes using each other's textbooks; we attend conferences to listen to each other speak on panels; we form committees among ourselves, and we tell the world the right answers. Nowhere in the process does the voice of Mr. Smith seem to play a role in how we conduct our business.
>
> Let Mr. Smith do one more thing. Let him stand outside the nursing home where Terri Schiavo lies. . . . Let Mr. Smith wave a picket sign, and declaim loudly to the television crews that experts like us are murdering Ms. Schiavo. At this point our bioethicists' interest in hearing Mr. Smith's voice reaches an all-time low Brody 2009:88-89.

I think that technocracy is illegitimate in a liberal democratic society. I share philosopher Michael Walzer's position that "it is a feature of democratic government that the people have a right to act wrongly" (Dzur and Levin 2004:335). If the citizens want to (stupidly, in some views) ban embryonic stem-cell research, then it is their right to do so. As Dzur and Levin summarize, "if democratic legitimacy means collective decisions by the individuals who are the subjects of those decisions, the role of the philosopher in a democracy cannot be to determine the proper results of those collective decisions" (Dzur and Levin 2004:335). As previously mentioned, Americans in particular will not accept of the idea that there is a profession that thinks it knows what the "true" values are, so a profession that explicitly claims this will not maintain jurisdiction.

It is the methods used by bioethicists that lead the profession toward technocracy. Common-morality principlism is not supposed to be technocratic, but due to the way that the specific principles of the American public are determined, it is. Like Brody's story, this technocracy increases as we move from health-care ethics consultation and research bioethics to public policy bioethics. We can at least conceivably craft a story about how the principles derived for research bioethics are those of the public. Recall that the principles were a philosophical back-filling of practices already used by scientists. So, for example, scientists had learned from exposure to the general public that individuals want to know if they are being experimented upon (autonomy), do not want to be harmed (nonmaleficence), and would ideally like to be helped (beneficence). Doctors working in hospitals probably figured out something similar over the years from interacting with patients. So, using the particular principles of the bioethics profession may be less technocratic in the research bioethics and health-care ethics consultation jurisdictions than in the public policy bioethics jurisdiction.

However, for the issues that are discussed in the public policy bioethics jurisdiction, like reproductive cloning and synthetic biology, there is no conceivable mechanism whereby the public's values are ascertained. Instead, the bioethics profession just extrapolates the values of the public in health-care ethics consultation and research bioethics to debates about public policy. The public has never been asked what its values are.

Of course, bioethicists have an explanation for how they know these particular principles represent the public's values, but the explanation strains credulity, and if publicized, would be unlikely to contribute to maintaining jurisdiction. Beauchamp and Childress claim to identify the common morality through reflection among academics about previous social disputes. Examples would be the Nuremberg trials or whatever social process led to the Hippocratic Oath (Engelhardt 2000:27). Beauchamp and Childress appear to follow W. D. Ross, who had "more influence on the present authors than any twentieth-century writer," when he claimed that "principles are 'recognized by intuitive induction as being implied in the judgments already passed on particular acts'" (Beauchamp and Childress 2001:402).

The method of academic reflection on major developments in Western history assumes that the issues that come to public prominence are those of most concern to the citizens, and these are resolved in a way that is consistent with what the public would want. This ignores the concept of power in history, however, whereby past disputes are often resolved in a way that makes them appear to be forwarding the interests of the general public, but are actually forwarding the interests of people with power. It ignores the oft-cited notion, probably most famously argued by Karl Marx, that the ruling ideas are the ideas of the ruling class. While I do not think a class analysis is particularly relevant to bioethical debate, the idea that the resolution of debates in history tells us much about the morality of *all* of the citizens—compared to the citizens with power—seems strained at best.

Ultimately, the advocates of the current common-morality principlism seem reluctant to let the public's values actually determine the principles. Beauchamp and Childress demonstrate this reluctance when they describe how they think the values of the public could be empirically determined. The principles should be empirically testable, they write, but they only want to include people in the empirical study who are already "committed to morality," which they have defined *a priori*. As they admit, some people will see this as tautological (Beauchamp and Childress 2009:393), and I am among the people who see it as such (Turner 2003:204). Their method of empirically determining the values or principles of the public suggests a reluctance to allow the public's values to drive bio-ethical conclusions, despite what bioethicists claim.

The bioethics profession's jurisdiction would be much stronger in public policy bioethics if they had a very clear and explicit claim that they should have jurisdiction because they represent the public's values. However, the technocratic impulse in the profession has pre-cluded credible demonstration of that claim. This is another feature of the bioethicists' system of abstract knowledge that must be modified.

Conclusion

In this chapter I began by clarifying the tasks in the task-spaces. The bioethics profession has worked out a quite effective subordi-nate jurisdictional settlement with the medical/scientific profession in the health-care ethics consultation and research bioethics juris-dictions wherein the bioethics profession does the work of enforc-ing the now-joint ethics of the medicine/science and bioethics professions. Bioethics also claims that its ethics are those of the public, which legitimates its ethical decisions. This subordinate jurisdiction is probably necessary in order for the profession to actu-ally do the task—you cannot be a watchdog from outside the fence.

The same subordinate jurisdiction, however, leads to difficulty in conducting the task in the public policy bioethics task-space, which must include the possibility of saying "no." The way that the task-spaces have been defined, how issues flow between them, the nature of the current principles, and other features lead to this tendency.

The profession would also have a stronger claim to jurisdiction if it made a justifiable argument for why it should be given this soapbox in the public square with which to influence policy. I argue against the use of a number of possible justifications and conclude that the current claim that bioethicists are representing the common morality is the most powerful. However, it is also not very credible, for despite claims to be representing the common morality, the profession seems to actually use a form of technocratic legitimation for its claims.

In the next chapter, I will suggest new methods for the system of abstract knowledge of the bioethics profession that will help defend the profession's jurisdictions. The new method will need to simultaneously maintain the subordinate jurisdictions in research bioethics and health-care ethics consultation, while breaking the subordinate jurisdiction in public policy bioethics and developing the ability to say "no." It will also much more clearly represent the common morality. I turn to this task next.

Notes

1. In my earlier work, I wrote that the bioethics profession had what Abbott labels an "advisory jurisdiction" with science wherein bioethics interpreted, buffered, or partially modified actions taken by science/medicine within science/medicine's own full jurisdiction (Abbott 1988:75). I no longer think this is quite right.

2. In Bosk's description, "bioethics developed within the institutional structure and with the institutional resources of academic medicine, and this undoubtedly influenced its critical thrust" (Bosk 1999:61).

3. Thanks to a reviewer from the press for reminding me of this point.

4. For an evaluation of these arguments, see Debruin (2007).

5. Conservative Protestants are defined following Steensland et al. (2000). Research has found that any existing religious conflict with science is generally not due to a dispute over epistemology (i.e., how truth is determined), but rather over values (Evans and Evans 2008; Evans and Evans 2010).

6. This point is a standard one in sociological analyses of principlism, perhaps because it is so classically sociological. Probably the first articulation of this critique was by Fox and Swazey (1984). See also, for example, DeVries and Subedi (1998).

Chapter 5

A Modified Method for the
Bioethics Profession

I *do* think that emerging technologies in science and medicine raise challenging ethical problems for society. I *do* think we need to find a way in the public sphere to discuss what we as a society should do about these technologies, and to forward that collective opinion to our elected officials. I *do* think there is a role for professional expertise in adjudicating between the general public and policy-makers. Ideally the ethics system used to recommend policy in public policy bioethics would also reflect the views of as many of the people in the country as possible. That is, I agree with the liberal impulse of forwarding the common morality that animated the first bioethicists. I also believe that bioethicists have a form of expertise in weighing and balancing societal values concerning scientific and medical issues, and that this expertise should be useful to government officials.

However, at present, the profession of bioethics is not up to for the task of recommending ethical policy because the methods used in its system of abstract knowledge lack legitimacy. Its jurisdiction in public policy bioethics is now threatened by social-movement activists, who are entirely willing to provide government officials with ethical advice. Its methods do not allow for the possibility of "no," and its powerful claim that it represents the public's views is not justified. This can be fixed. All professions modify their system of abstract knowledge to make them more functional over time, and it is simply time that the profession of bioethics made some improvements.

I suspect that if we were to look at the history of the professions, radical change is extremely rare, and that incremental change is the dominant process. What I am advocating in this chapter is incrementalist; the underlying logic of the system of abstract knowledge of the bioethics profession would not change. Bioethicists would also still be writing journal articles, teaching, consulting, and everything else that they currently do in three of the four jurisdictions. The profession would still be representing the values of others. In general, what is required is a greater attention to the different tasks in the three task-spaces bioethicists are claiming jurisdiction in and, in particular, a much closer focus on the methods used by the profession.

A New Method for the Public Policy Bioethics Jurisdiction

Again, I do think the first bioethicists had the right idea in claiming that through advancing the common morality they represented all the citizens, because such a claim, if legitimate, would be a powerful argument for jurisdiction. However, the consensus among diverse commissioners method is not going to work. The very concept has been too de-legitimized, given that the right and then the left so forcefully made the case that the existing ethics commissions were not representative of the public's views. As an example, in 2007, Trotter wrote, "for a consensus of bioethicists to bear authority for public policy decisions in a pluralistic democracy like the United States, it would need to be connected in some demonstrable way to the moral intuitions and considered judgements of the general population. Such a connection is not manifest when selected samples of uniformly leftward bioethicists convene on panels such as the National Bioethics Advisory Commission" (Trotter 2007:114). Liberals would of course fire back that the connection is also not manifest by the more right-leaning President's Council on Bioethics of the George W. Bush era.

To defend their jurisdiction from the social-movement activists, bioethicists need to quite explicitly and quite loudly use their form of democratic legitimacy as a weapon, saying in effect that "we are representing the values of the entire public, not some special interest, like the social movements are." This is actually saying that bioethicists are more qualified to conduct the task in the task-space, namely, recommending ethical policy that will be applied to all citizens. The bioethics profession currently hides its justifications, and it takes an expert to ferret out that it is actually claiming to represent the entire citizenry. I speculate that the reason it does not currently discuss the justification for its jurisdiction is either that members of the profession do not actually believe they represent the values of the public, they want to promote their own values, or they are fearful that they will not be taken seriously in these divisive times for loudly claiming there is a universal morality. However, if their methods of deriving the common morality can be improved, then they can feel less shy about advertising their qualifications for the task in the jurisdiction.

Take the Human Embryo Research Panel as an example, whose ethical recommendations were rejected by President Clinton, and whose proposals were later explicitly legislated against by Congress. To its religious-right critics, it reached the wrong ethical conclusions about embryos, and these religious-right activists clearly had the ear of all of these elected officials who rejected the bioethics profession's conclusions. While the Panel tried to make it clear that they were not speaking for themselves, but for the general public, their methods were not convincing enough that they could use them to support their ethical recommendations. What if the methods used by the bioethics profession much more clearly represented the values of the public? Bioethicists could then say that their religious-right adversaries were putting their own values above those of the public, and President Clinton himself was doing the same. Will this stop religious-right activists from saying that embryos should still not be killed, even if the public thinks differently? Of course not, but it will give the bioethics profession a much more powerful argument against these competitors from social movements.

A Reformed Common-Morality Principlism

Bioethics needs to retain the claim of representing the common morality, but using methods that are convincing enough that they can loudly say that their ethical recommendations are better than their competitors' because they are representing the public. They also need to be able to say "no," because that is part of the task in public policy bioethics. We are left with the job of reforming common-morality principlism.

The first problem with principlism that makes its connection to the actual common morality of the public unclear is that is that the principles themselves are vague. Critics have pointed out that this vagueness means that one can reach any ethical conclusion with the same principles (Harris 2003:306). As Leigh Turner notes, "[a]greement at the level of general norms has no inherent practical significance since it is possible to derive markedly divergent policies and practices from the 'same' principle, maxim, or moral intuition." For example, "[o]ne person can use the principles to make the case for the legalization of physician-assisted suicide, while another individual can argue that physician-assisted suicide should never be legalized." This then means that for "the principles to have meaning and weight, they require interpretation," which then "requires some substantive commitments" (Turner 2003:195–196).

Much of the ethical action happens in the specification of principles, and this specification is done with reference to the particular value community of the analyst, not of the public. This makes the application of principles appear to not be based on universal values at all. Therefore, we need principles that are less vague.

The first step toward creating principles that are less vague, and therefore more closely reflect the public's values, is to redefine the term *common* in *common morality*. Bioethicists mean by this the few values that are "common to everyone," as in "universal." But of course this is rhetorical. For example, not everyone in the United States holds autonomy as a principle. We could imagine that 99% believe in beneficence and non-maleficence, 80% in autonomy, and 75% in justice. Rejecting the rhetorical claim to universality, the profession should explicitly state a level of acceptance of a principle before it is considered "universal enough" to represent the common morality. Skipping how this would be determined for a moment, let us just set 80% as a placeholder. Therefore, a principle is held in a high degree of consensus in American society if 80% of the people adhere to it. So, step one is to acknowledge that there are no universal principles in the United States, but to explicitly say that principles with a high degree of consensus will be used to recommend ethical policy for the public.

This is not anti-democratic. Idiosyncratic extremists who do not have the same values as everyone else are never given veto power in liberal democratic societies. (The exception is a Constitutional claim, and I do not think any bioethical issues reach that level.)[1] I, for one, am quite used to the idea that my idiosyncratic ethics are almost entirely unrepresented among policy-makers, but I do not think the democratic system is less legitimate for this fact, but rather I conclude that I have to persuade more people in the public sphere to share my ethics. Similarly, Quakers know their values are ignored in public debates, and know they need to convince more people to adhere to them before they will be considered a legitimate perspective. So, if principles do not have to be so vague that they are shared by 100% of the population, but only 80%, we have made the first step toward principles that would be specific enough to influence policy recommendations.

The greatest source of vagueness that makes the connection to the common morality unclear enters with the fact that the current version of principlism is based on transmutation, not condensed translation. In transmutation, rich ethical concerns of the public are examined, and only the part that can fit with the four existing principles is accepted as an argument, even if this accepted part is quite peripheral to the heart of the public's concern. Unaccepted parts of the argument are discarded. For example, "playing God" with genetic engineering was transmuted to concerns about the risk that a modified life form could damage the environment. This makes it appear that the citizenry's concerns are not being addressed. In condensed translation, the core of the concern is simplified but accurate, and translations will appear to represent the original concern. My reformed principlism will be based on condensed translations, not transmutations. It will take the debate back to the second era wherein participants in the debate examined the technology in question and created condensed and secular translations of their values for a pluralistic debate. So, instead of squeezing an ethical debate into institutionalized principles or values that can be used for any issue, a debate would start by asking what the principles or values of the public *are* for the issue. This would also make the principles less vague because they would be related to the issue at hand.

If we are to start with a technology, and see what American values are regarding that technology, bioethicists are also going to have to abandon the idea that the principles are universal across all issues. Both the claim that the principles are universally shared by all people and the claim that the principles are universal across all issues are the result of the bioethics profession's ignoring who actually confers jurisdiction. In the 1970s bioethics was a new enterprise whose academic status was shaky at best. It needed to have academic credibility in order to be a part of the modern university, given that its proponents worked in universities, not for the state. Both the cross-person and the cross-issue universalism would have served to bolster the legitimacy of principlism in the eyes of academic philosophy. Moreover, many of the early theoreticians of principlism were trained as analytic philosophers.

Analytic philosophy, perhaps ultimately because of Enlightenment commitments, but not necessarily for my argument, has a commitment to universal theories. As Howard Brody summarizes, analytic philosophy argues that "any true ethical statement ought to take the form of a universal proposition that holds for all cultures and all historical periods," and "Anglo-American analytical philosophy, for much of the twentieth century, treated universality as a *sine qua non* of ethics" (Brody 2009:117, 212). Believing in universal moral principles is then a minimum for principlists to create a system that was unified enough to pass muster with the philosophical community. However, this concern of philosophers is not relevant to operating as a profession in the public sphere, as the American Philosophical Association does not provide jurisdiction over public policy bioethics. I recognize that my new method may cause professional philosophers to think less of the profession of bioethics, which may cause trouble for bioethicists ensconced in philosophy departments.

So, the bioethics profession would give up both universal claims—that four principles are universally applicable to all medical and scientific issues, and that these principles or values are universally held by all persons. These changes result in the following: If we think in terms of principles, there may be a common morality about human experimentation or health-care issues that is represented in principles A, B, C, and D, which are held by 80% of the population. With issues in public policy bioethics, the values of the public regarding human genetic engineering might be represented by A, C, E, F, and H. With cloning, the public's values may be represented by A, E, and J.

Evidence suggests that some members of the bioethics profession, while not really having explicitly thought through this issue, have at least implicitly accepted abandoning both universal claims. For example, the Advisory Committee on Human Radiation Experiments of the Clinton presidency, active in the mid-1990s, had many prominent bioethicists as commissioners and used the system of abstract knowledge of the bioethics profession. The task at hand was to review the ethics of U.S. government radiation experimentation on people during the Cold War—experimentation that often occurred without the people's consent or sometimes even knowledge.

In their final report, they note that "the Advisory Committee is in essence a national ethics commission" (Advisory Committee on Human Radiation Experiments 1996:113). In keeping with the system of abstract knowledge of bioethicists, they note the central problem of moral pluralism, and use as a central component of their moral evaluation "basic ethical principles that are widely accepted and generally regarded as so fundamental as to be applicable to the past as well as the present." Here the standard is not "universal" but "widely accepted and generally regarded." Then, reflecting the fact that the profession has not thought this through, this is closely followed by a universal statement that "basic ethical principles are general standards or rules that all morally serious individuals accept" (Advisory Committee on Human Radiation Experiments 1996:114). (Ignoring some citizens in the evaluation of the universal morality due to these citizens' lack of moral seriousness seems to be how bioethics theoreticians deal with the fact that there is no perfect moral consensus about any value.)

While open a bit to non-universality across persons, more importantly they seem to have engaged in condensed translation, not transmutation, to obtain principles different from those used for other issues in bioethical debates, reporting that they identified not four, but "six basic ethical principles as particularly relevant to our work." These included: "One ought not to treat people as mere means to the ends of others"; "One ought not to deceive others"; "One ought not to inflict harm or risk of harm"; "One ought to promote welfare and prevent harm"; "One ought to treat people fairly and with equal respect"; and "One ought to respect the self-determination of others" (Advisory Committee on Human Radiation Experiments 1996:114).

This embodies my plan. Despite some contradictory statements, the principles are not thought to be universal—principles do not need to be made so vague that neo-Nazis are included in the consensus. More important, through condensed translation the principles more closely fit the concerns of the public regarding this particular issue. The actual values of the public do not need to be transmuted into the ill-fitting principles of autonomy, beneficence, non-maleficence, and justice. Ethical conclusions based on weighing and balancing these principles are more likely to be recognized as representing the values of the citizens, increasing the odds of the bioethics profession's retaining jurisdiction over public policy bioethics.

A New Public Policy Bioethics Jurisdictional Settlement

However, as is standard for the profession, the Advisory Committee did not reveal how they identified the principles, and I suspect it was done through academic reflection by the commissioners and staff. This particular method of condensed translation is never going to overcome the suspicion that the condensed values are actually those of the bioethicists, not the public. Therefore, to avoid the perception of technocracy, bioethicists will have to engage in an advisory jurisdiction with the profession of social science to determine what the common morality of most of the citizens is for each issue. This will be an extremely modest trimming of the bioethicists' jurisdiction in that almost no work is actually done by bioethicists in the area they would be giving up. Bioethicists usually just assert the values or principles of the public. As we saw in the introduction, bioethics does not even claim that measuring the values of the public is something they do.

My recommended role for social science in bioethical debate is very limited compared to the recommendations of my fellow social scientists, who have made many criticisms of the bioethics profession in general and common-morality principlism in particular (Bosk 1999; Hedgecoe 2004; Fox and Swazey 2008; DeVries and Subedi 1998; Turner 2009; Salter and Jones 2005; Yearley 2009; Belkin 2004). To take but one example, Charles Bosk notes that social scientists seek out the sort of context for ethical decisions that principlism tries to ignore. Social scientists tend to ask how a "problem" comes to be seen as "ethical" in the first place, which is where most of the sociological action is, and not how it is later "resolved" (Bosk 1999). The social science version of bioethics is largely incompatible with bioethics as it is currently practiced. Again, Bosk is worth quoting at length:

> In a very real way, if ethnographies of medical settings are properly done, they may very well cut against the objectives of bioethicists. There may be a built-in incompatibility between bioethical and sociological inquiry, and heightening this tension rather than attempting to deny it may very well be a useful contribution of the social scientist to bioethics. . . . The goal of social science, especially as practiced by ethnographers (again, this is my assumption), is to show how actors shape and trim their actions to fit their principles and how these same actors shape and trim their values and principles to fit their actions. Where bioethicists seek clarity, social scientists look for ambiguity and complexity (Bosk 1999:65).

Moreover, there has been much discussion of how social science research can inform ethics by theoreticians of the emerging field of empirical bioethics (DeVries and Gordijn 2009; Leget, Borry and DeVries 2009; Hedgecoe 2004; Borry, Schotsmans and Dierickx 2005). There is very little agreement about how to even describe this debate, and many typologies of the possible relationships between social science and bioethics exist. My proposal is so mild that it verges on what Ray DeVries has labeled "sociology in bioethics"—sociology in the service of a master discipline (DeVries 2003). For example, a central question in this emerging debate is whether the use of social science for ethics would generate an "is/ ought" problem (DeVries and Gordijn 2009). Simply, philosophers hold that you cannot derive an "ought" (infanticide is wrong) from an "is" (everyone thinks infanticide is wrong.) The classic objection is that few white people in the eighteenth century thought that slavery was wrong, so you should not derive an "ought" from an "is." Much of the interesting work of the theoreticians of empirical bioethics is to find a way to incorporate empiricism into our normative analysis.

However, my recommended method does not even invoke the "is/ought" problem. It is only in public policy ethics where I want to follow the values of the public—as should be expected in a democracy. In cultural bioethics, we should most definitively *not* allow the "is" to determine the "ought." Rather, outside of the realm of government policy, people should try to convince others about what our ethics should be regardless of what people currently believe. Even the philosophically inclined bioethicists themselves think we should be following the values or principles of the public in public policy bioethics, so I am not even threatening this basic distinction.

In my professional-jurisdiction language, a social science that tries to create a new epistemological foundation for the ethical analysis of medicine and science would have to engage in a frontal attempt to strip jurisdiction from the bioethicists. And, indeed, much of the social science critique of bioethics has this quality. However, it is not that the social scientists are wrong, but rather they are unrealistic in that their critique does not acknowledge that something like a common-morality principlism is necessary for research bioethics, health-care ethics consultation, and public policy bioethics. To use sociological lingo, there are structural features of the public sphere and the state that select for common-morality principlism, as I showed in previous chapters.

Therefore, instead of a revolutionary solution of my colleagues, I propose a reformist one. Principlism is here to stay. It fits with the way bureaucracies work, it is easily calculable and applicable by part-time bioethicists. It is semitransparent and can accurately depict the general values of the public. However, for the bioethics profession to have legitimacy, I propose the empirical derivation of common-morality principles through a form of condensed translation.

Empirical Measurement of Principles

Political theorists John S. Dryzek and Simon Niemeyer have recently offered an interesting proposal that democracies be designed for the representation of discourses, not necessarily the representation of persons (Dryzek and Niemeyer 2008). They even recommend a "Chamber of Discourses," which would be "a small issue-specific deliberating group that contains representatives of all relevant discourses" in a society (Dryzek and Niemeyer 2008:485). They would effectively be put in a room and told to come up with a solution to a problem (like a regular legislature that represents individuals is currently told to do).

They argue that representing discourses is just as democratically legitimate as representing persons, because the person-model does not represent a person *per se*, but rather their interests, identities and values. We are all "multiple selves" who use some discourses and not others. Since it is our interests, values, and so on that are represented in the person-representation model, why not just directly represent the interests and values (what they call "discourses") themselves? They conclude that: "once we accept the insight from discursive psychology that any individual may engage multiple discourses, it is important that all these discourses get represented. Otherwise, the individual in his or her entirety is not represented. Discursive representation may, then, do a morally superior [or a][2] more comprehensive job of representing persons than do theories that treat individuals as unproblematic wholes" (Dryzek and Niemeyer 2008:483).

I do not want to replace Congress with a Chamber of Discourses. However, if we substitute their term *discourses*, for the more common bioethics term *principles*, or *values*, you can see my analogy, which is that their Chamber of Discourses is a model for my new version of a government ethics commission that can make recommendations about policy to Congress or to the Executive Branch. The first step is to determine the principles that must be represented. Dryzek and Niemeyer outline many standard social science methods that can and have been used for this task, such as historical analysis of public discourse, in-depth interviews, focus groups, and opinion surveys.

This is all standard fare in the social sciences. The authors describe a study of Russian society that identifies three discourses (chastened democracy, reactionary anti-liberalism, authoritarian development). They describe a study of U.S. environmental politics that identifies seven. Another study of criminal justice finds four in the public (psychopathology of criminals, rational choice, social causes of crime, social dislocation of individual offenders) (Dryzek and Niemeyer 2008:487).

I have conducted a study of the discourses that religious Americans use to discuss reproductive genetic technologies (Evans 2010). Typical of the social sciences, I began with an in-depth qualitative study that examined a not-exactly-representative group of religious Americans. This inductive analysis provided an initial window into how citizens think about an issue, and initial conclusions were made. I also used a nationally representative survey that was representative of the people in the country. This could easily be repeated for the public at large.

Social science certainly thinks it can engage in condensed translation, as it does so all the time, as shown by the endless stream of books about the limited number of discourses used by a group. For example, Bellah and his colleagues in *Habits of the Heart*, one of the most influential sociology books of all time, found four moral languages in use in the United States (Bellah et al. 1985).

Moreover, it is a premise of the emerging field of *empirical bioethics* that this is possible (DeVries and Gordijn 2009:193).

I agree with Dryzek and Niemeyer that triangulation between multiple methods would be desirable (Dryzek and Niemeyer 2008:487). Analogous with the abandonment of the idea of universality across persons, rarely used principles would be excluded, which would make the ethical analysis richer, because a radically thin "lowest common denominator" would not be required.

Some issues are too new either for people to have thought about or for any discourse in the public sphere to really exist—yet a decision about them needs to be made now. For example, if a public policy bioethics body wanted to make an ethical recommendation about synthetic biology—where life forms are created *de novo*—it needs to be done now, before there is time for an extensive public debate. There are many solutions to this problem, usually focused upon citizens' learning facts about the technology before they discuss the ethics of it. For example, deliberative-democracy advocates (Gutmann and Thompson 1996) cite many examples of deliberative processes, such as the 1990 Oregon Health Plan public deliberations and deliberative polling.[3]

Dryzek and Niemeyer want to evaluate discourses. In social science, there is a distinction between *discourse*, what I am calling *values* or *ends*, and what bioethicists would call *principles*. I recognize that bioethicists do not like equating principles with values or ends, because in their precise theoretical formulations they *are* different. I believe that while values/ends and principles may in theory be different, in the hands of an ordinary bioethicist they are the same, and the ability of social science to discriminate between them is limited. (However, it is never stated how bioethicists tell the difference using their method of academic reflection.) Since advocates of principlism claim that things called "principles" are held by the public, social scientists would consult with bioethicists to make sure they are measuring the principles that bioethicists want as their raw material, not the (closely) related discourses, values, or ends.

In fact, bioethicists already extensively use social science research in their work, such as studies to see if normative problems exist. For example, the President's Commission of the early 1980s conducted an empirical study of hospital ethics committees (President's Commission for the Study of Ethical Problems in Medicine and Biomedical and Behavioral Research 1983a). The profession of bioethics also generally supports the burgeoning field of "empirical bioethics" that uses social science methodology to examine, for example, what people really think they are doing when they sign informed-consent forms. Bioethics commissions have even commissioned social science research on the attitudes or values of the public, although they have not been clear how such data inform their ethical recommendations. The first bioethics commission conducted an empirical study of people's views of the implications of advances in biomedical and behavioral research (National Commission for the Protection of Human Subjects of Biomedical and Behavioral Research 1978b), and the President's Commission of the early 1980s conducted a survey of the general public's views of informed consent in the doctor–patient interaction (President's Commission for the Study of Ethical Problems in Medicine and Biomedical and Behavioral Research 1982). With regard to the empirical measurement of principles, Beauchamp and Childress have themselves acknowledged that their four principles should be empirically verifiable with social science (Beauchamp and Childress 2009:393–94).[4]

Note that in this system, the structures of principlism that make it more difficult to say "no" have been removed. The principles for public policy bioethics and research bioethics would not be the same, so describing an issue with principles in public policy bioethics will not automatically make the issue fall under the jurisdiction of research bioethics. While the empirically derived principles for research bioethics and health-care ethics consultation would probably remain individualistic (i.e., autonomy), there is no reason why issues in the public policy bioethics jurisdiction would be so.

For example, I think the public will have collectively oriented principles for anything having to do with the nature of humans, such as with genetics.

In sum, the new form of principlism would be less vague because each issue would have its own principles, and the principles would be more explicitly derived from the values of the public. They would not always point to "yes," as the current principles do in public policy bioethics. These changes would allow for the bioethics profession to be more convincing to the jurisdiction-givers in public policy bioethics—government officials—that it was representing the public's values and thus was the most qualified profession to have jurisdiction over the task of suggested policies that will be applied to *all* citizens. This will help in its competition with the social-movement activists.

Objections

One complaint could be that I have just described the Sociologist Full Employment Act. However there are enough medical sociologists and anthropologists currently working in bioethics centers to do this task, so there would be no spike in the employment of social science Ph.D.s. People could also object that the results will be fuzzy. The values that the citizens want to advance through scientific and medical technology will be difficult to describe, and they will to some extent be contradictory. This complaint can be dismissed by the adage about the drunk looking for his lost keys under the lamppost because that is where the light is. You cannot only ask the easy ethical questions. Instead, the standard of evaluation should be: Is this a better way of determining the common morality than what we currently have? I would argue that the current method is academic reflection on what the analyst thinks the public morality is.[5] This method would have to be better, if for no other reason than that there is a record of how the analysts came to their conclusions.

Moreover, remember that we are gauging the citizens' principles or values so they can be used as inputs to elite debate. Judgement will still be required. The bioethical commission would have that task, and it will undoubtedly be more difficult when their raw material is the *actual* conflicting principles of the American people. And of course we should remember that our society currently sets policy based on evaluating the values of the public through far less precise methods. As a summary of sociological analysis of studies of actual forms of political representation in the public sphere reminds us, "it is crucial to recognize that any mechanism for translating preferences into policy must systematically distort, refract, magnify, and distill those preferences in various ways" (Perrin and McFarland 2008:1239).

For example, the structural mechanism for the expression of our values in public affairs is the elected official who is supposed to represent the values of his or her constituents. It would take a large leap of faith to describe the electoral system as accurately doing this. Similarly, in some states, policy is determined through ballot initiatives. Not only does an initiative become policy if only 50% plus one of the citizens vote for it, but the way the citizens are informed of the issues borders on systematic and deliberate misinformation campaigns. Social science would be at least as good at determining the public's values as would either of these methods, and it would certainly have to be better than the current method of scholarly reflection.

Will the public be convinced that this new method measures ordinary values? The public is not so familiar with how social science could determine which principles are used for an issue. For example, the public does not necessarily understand how a random selection can be used to determine a representative sample of a larger entity. Dryzek and Niemeyer have a number of solutions to this problem, such as making sure that the social science itself is conducted as democratically and transparently as possible. The social science could involve citizens themselves, with social scientists as consultants, and all of the data could be available for public viewing. Of course, some residual distrust would remain, but it would certainly be more accurate and transparent than the method of determining the public's principles currently used by bioethicists.

The Task of Bioethics Professionals

To be clear, for my new version of public policy bioethics, social science would empirically determine the values or principles used in society, and then bioethicists would do what bioethicists who use principlism are good at—weighing and balancing conflicting principles and determining if the means in question (e.g., human genetic engineering) maximizes those principles.

Dryzek and Niemeyer advocate that any one commissioner represent one or two discourses in their Chamber of Discourses. In the analogous public policy bioethics commission, without assigned principles, it would be easy for the group to technocratically decide that some of the principles of the public are beyond the pale, not legitimate enough for consideration in any ethical recommendation. For example, at present I think most liberal bioethicists would not believe in a principle such as "we should keep the basic constitution of humans like it is now." Yet, I would imagine that this would be a principle that would be identified through social science if the issue were, for example, genetic science. Therefore, bioethicists would be selected to be on the commission to represent principles they believe in. Dryzek and Niemeyer describe a methodology to find representatives who load heavily on one discourse (Dryzek and Niemeyer 2008:486).

The jurisdiction of the bioethics profession over public policy bioethics would then continue as it does now, but in modified form. The morality of the public expressed as principles would be determined by social scientists. Once the principles had been determined, how these principles on each issue were balanced, weighed, and, most important, connected to the scientific or medical practice or issue, would remain in the hands of the bioethics profession. This is where bioethical expertise comes in. To take but one example: let us say we can determine five principles that the public would like to maximize when it comes to human genetic engineering. That we have come up with five and not one suggests we are getting somewhat specific, moving away from vagueness. That we have come up with five and not ten reflects the limited cognitive capacities of humans in that no bioethicist could relate ten principles to each other in one analysis. With these five values or principles in hand, what ethical policy do we then suggest for germline human genetic engineering? What if the hypothetical value of "autonomy" clashes with the hypothetical value of "keeping humans like we have always been." This is a bioethical dilemma, but it is a less technocratic dilemma than one that specifies, balances, and weighs values that have not been shown to be held by the public on whose behalf policies are being suggested. This new method would be harder for critics of the bioethics profession to criticize, because the de-legitimators would have a harder time arguing that bioethicists are simply using their own values.

Dryzek and Niemeyer are not advocating that the Chamber of Discourses necessarily replace a body that represents individuals (like the U.S. Congress). It could be advisory—as an additional form of input for the government representatives who must make policy, just like public policy bioethics is now. So analogously, in my proposal, the new version of the bioethics commission would be like the old, proposing ethical policy to elected officials, albeit with a stronger claim to be articulating the values of the public. The public could still debate and communicate their desires with elected officials through social movements, political activism, and elections. This dual track of input to government officials is therefore also unchanged from the existing situation.

Of course, public policy bioethics is not solely composed of government ethics commissions, and many other bioethicists would want to make policy recommendations. If they are going to be writing about suggested policy using their bioethics-profession identity, they will need to use the empirically derived principles of the public as their base, acting as their own bioethics commission. They can debate the best conclusion to reach from the public's values. Bioethics would be even more clearly perceived as the profession that makes ethical policy suggestions based on the public's principles or values on each issue in science and medicine. They would use this perception to defend their jurisdiction.

Is This Not Technocratic?

On the surface, this proposal violates my injunction against technocracy, where experts rule. However, opposition to technocracy is not opposition to technical experts, but rather the substitution of their values for the public's values through the claim of expertise. In my system, unlike the old, the public's values are represented. My system is somewhat technocratic, in that the link between the means (i.e., a technology) and the ends (public values) would be determined by experts. This is the component of the ethical decision that *is* the most technical, so I do not see my proposal as usurping the role of the public.

That said, my proposal will not convince someone who was opposed to the existence of public policy bioethics in the first place. Such a person would ask: why not simply have the public deliberate on, not only their values, but whether a technological means fits with their values, and then forward their views to their elected officials. In an ideal liberal democratic public sphere, I agree that such a proposal would be best.

However, we do not have an ideal public sphere. There are so many vested interests with power and money influencing how public discourse operates that any debate is systematically distorted. Anyone can give myriad examples, but the recurring debates over health-care policy in America seem to me at least to be subject to incredible distortion by groups with money, where they zero in on actual public values, and then distort descriptions of the means (various specific policies) so that the means seem to violate the public's values. An example is the claim that the Obama administration's health-care reform will result in the euthanasia of children with Down syndrome. I have no doubt the vast majority of the public would hold a value that led to opposing euthanizing children with Down syndrome, but the connection of this means (a new health-care system) to that value strikes me as totally false, promoted by people with power and interests in the public sphere.

Another problem with our actual public sphere is that communication seems to be increasingly stratified. When I was a child, before cable television, there were four television channels, but now there are hundreds, each with its own perspective on the world. Viewers of Fox News and MSNBC exist in distinct discursive worlds, and the values in the two worlds will be unlikely to encounter each other. Discussion across moral worlds is difficult, but it would occur by design in the new public policy bioethics. While some flattening of moral values would occur in the data-reduction of the social science, truly polarized values would both be represented (e.g., "pro-choice/pro-life").

Of course, public policy bioethics will not replace the public sphere. It would simply be a resource for policy-makers to refer to see how a group of experts separated from the severest constraints of the public sphere come to conclusions about medical or scientific technologies and practices in light of the public's values.

The End of Public Policy Bioethics' Subsidiary Jurisdiction to Science/Medicine in

One drawback to my plan is that while it would probably retain the subsidiary jurisdiction with medicine and science in the research bioethics and health-care ethics consultation task-spaces, it may make the science and medicine professions opposed to the bioethics profession in public policy bioethics. The science/medicine profession may well continue the current version of principlism or come up with its own ethics to compete with the bioethicists.

The divorce may come as the bioethics profession starts saying "no" much more often. Obviously, this is a reason why it would be more difficult to implement my reforms, because the profession of bioethics could get thrown out of the house of medicine. However, without reforms, if bioethics as a profession is totally de-legitimized, it will eventually be thrown out of the house for being useless. Unfortunately, bioethics is not going to benefit from social science in the new jurisdictional relationship wherein social science is the subsidiary and bioethics is the master profession. To put it crudely, social science has only a tiny fraction of the wealth and power that the medical and scientific professions control, so bioethicists would not want to depend upon it for resources.

The Research Bioethics Subsidiary Jurisdiction

I now turn to my suggestions for the other jurisdictions the profession of bioethics competes for. As noted above, the bioethics profession's subsidiary jurisdiction in research bioethics seems secure, and while I have not examined whether this is true, it is plausible that the current common-morality principlist system of abstract knowledge used by the bioethics profession actually does roughly represent the common morality on this one issue. This makes sense because it was designed for exactly this purpose, and only later was extrapolated to other issues and other jurisdictions. The designers of the principles *for use in research bioethics* actually had some informal social data in the form of the scientists' practices that had been shaped by fear of public reaction to research scandals. For example, the principle of autonomy was extrapolated from the existing practice of informed consent, which was solidified by scientists long before bioethics came into being, out of fear that the public might react negatively to a scandal. From this they found out that people wanted to give their own permission to be in a research study, did not want to be hurt, and so on.

That said, eventually there should be an empirical confirmation that the current principles *are* the public's values for human research. There are some hints that principlism may not represent the public's values in research bioethics. For example, Oonagh Corrigan found that, in clinical drug trials, the ethical focus is on autonomy and informed consent, but this "ignores factors which are vitally important to patients, simply because they are external to the concept of autonomy" (in Hedgecoe 2004:127).

The jurisdiction-giver for the joint science/medicine/bioethics jurisdiction over research bioethics remains the federal government. Social movements seem unconcerned with research bioethics. As I have articulated in previous chapters, a system of abstract knowledge based on maximizing fixed commensurable principles is necessary for the sorts of bureaucratic contexts that this ethics operates in. Presuming that the four principles as currently articulated *are* the values of American society *for the issues of human experimentation*, then the subsidiary jurisdiction of bioethicists is also democratically legitimate. It would not be the ethics only of some particular interest group, nor is it technocratic; again, assuming that these are the values of the public that are being maximized. No changes are necessary.

The Health-Care Ethics Consultation Subsidiary Jurisdiction

The bioethics profession's subsidiary jurisdiction with science/ medicine over health-care ethics consultation also seems secure. Here jurisdiction is given by a complex combination of hospital bureaucrats, the general public, and, increasingly, the bureaucratic state via the oversight of hospital regulatory agencies and the courts. Principlism seems dominant and appropriate, and the current principles (without using the principle of justice) are probably a good fit with the values that the public would like to use in health-care ethics. No change is needed, and with research bioethics, this jurisdiction forms the core of the jurisdictional homeland of the bioethics profession.

However, the bioethics profession is trying to expand its jurisdiction to tasks adjacent to health-care ethics consultation, and it is here that, without solidifying the methods in their system of abstract knowledge, the profession's seemingly secure jurisdiction may be damaged. The professional association of bioethicists has previously written that health-care ethics consultation should mediate between the values and ethics of the various parties to a medical decision, such as family members, doctors, and the hospital administration, but only allowing options that are "ethically justifiable and consistent with prevailing ethical and legal standards" (American Society for Bioethics and Humanities 2011:12). There is no discussion about how those involved with health-care ethics consultation are supposed to determine what the "prevailing ethics" are, besides an examination of the bioethical literature, statements of bioethics commissions, and so forth. Textbooks used to teach health-care ethics consultation imply that principlism is the source of "prevailing ethics."

This is of course what a profession with strongly institutionalized jurisdiction would do. For example, medicine can simply say that doctors must act in a way consistent with medical knowledge and be done with it. However, bioethics is not that strong. If and when a bioethicist claims that the desires of the family or the desires of the hospital administration are not consistent with "prevailing ethics," someone is going to challenge how the "prevailing ethics" was determined. At present, I would argue that there is not an answer that would be acceptable or even understandable to the public. Empirically determining the principles of the public for health-care ethics consultation would provide a justification for "prevailing ethics."

More critically, the bioethics profession is in the midst of simultaneously trying to shore up this jurisdiction and to expand it, increasingly claiming that it is not only the ethics "by the bedside" that is under its jurisdiction, but the ethics of the hospital as an organization (Slowther 2007). The bioethicists' association report on core competencies for health-care ethics consultation "endorses the trend toward integrating ethics across all subspecialties in an organization," which includes business, professional, and organizational ethics (American Society for Bioethics and Humanities 2011:5). If the profession continues down this path, it will encounter people with much greater power who will have the resources to challenge the basis of the profession's ethics if faced with a recommendation they do not like. It would be useful for the profession to have backed up the claims that principlism represents the public's values regarding human experimentation and ethical decisions in hospitals before claiming that their ethics can also inform the business decisions of the hospital.

Cultural Bioethics

Finally, I call for the bioethics profession to abandon its work in the cultural bioethics jurisdiction. In cultural bioethics, professionals try to persuade the ordinary citizens of the fitness of a particular ethical stance in relation to a scientific/medical technology or practice, independent of policy proposals. It is in this sphere that the general public should be having an extensive debate about science and medicine. Ideally, every religious congregation, social club, and dinner party would have citizens deliberating about the ethics of technologies like reproductive cloning. Professionals forward particular arguments into this public sphere that citizens adopt, build upon, criticize, or ignore. This shaping clearly happens, as citizens now seem to make a moral distinction between "reproductive" and "therapeutic" cloning—a distinction advocated by professionals in cultural bioethics, speaking through the institutions of the public sphere like the media.

Contributions to Cultural Bioethics by Non-Bioethicists

All professionals but bioethicists—and any citizen—should make the argument for and against some technology or practice (a means) *and* for or against some moral value or principle. The current level of acceptance of the claims by the public is irrelevant—perhaps the idiosyncratic views are even more important to debate in order to shake things up. Theologians can argue for the value of obeying God, and that germline-enhancement human genetic engineering would be disobeying God. Philosophers can argue for maximizing human happiness, and that human genetic engineering is a means that forwards this end. Transhumanists can argue for human self-perfection through human genetic engineering. Such claims are critical for the health of the public sphere and for democracy in general, as we must have a debate about what we value and how to achieve our values. Not debating our ends or values, and only debating the most efficacious means toward assumed or undebatable ends, has long been the subject of social critique (Evans 2002:13). Participants in bioethical debate have been similarly concerned. Nearly 40 years ago, Leon Kass, in criticizing participants in the bioethical debate about genetics who did not want to debate our ends or principles, wrote the following vignette:

> Good afternoon, ladies and gentlemen. This is your pilot speaking. We are flying at an altitude of 35,000 feet and a speed of 700 miles an hour. I have two pieces of news to report, one good and one bad. The bad news is that we are lost. The good news is that we are making very good time.[6]

Society was "flying" toward perfecting the means to modify the human genome, but we did not know why we were doing so. "We are told that new technologies are coming and that we should attend, consider, and adjust to the social consequences," Kass wrote. However, "this formulation treats new developments as automatic, as insensitive to human decision and choice. But only a slavish mind and a slavish society let the means dictate the ends."[7] In sum, we have to have the debate about what our ends should be in cultural bioethics.

Nobody should be using any form of common-morality principlism in cultural bioethics, as this would simply reinforce current values. Finally, if you only want to advocate "true" or "correct" values, then you belong in cultural bioethics, not in the other jurisdictions. Bioethicists become more like lawyers who are not supposed to evaluate the guilt or innocence of their clients, but rather have a role in representing them effectively.

Obviously the ends or principles reached by the public in the broader public sphere (cultural bioethics) influence public policy bioethics in my proposed system, albeit with a time lag. For example, if proponents of utilitarianism in cultural bioethics come to convince more and more people that the most important value is human happiness, then more and more of the public will want to be maximizing utility through medical and scientific interventions. This change in public's views would show up in the next round of social science analysis of the principles of the public. In turn, this would influence public policy bioethics, with recommended policies' being slightly more influenced by this type of thought.

Contributions to Cultural Bioethics by "Bioethicists"

Again, bioethicists, acting as professional bioethicists, should abandon cultural bioethics. Bioethicists would be, under my system, the professionals whose system of abstract knowledge is to represent the public's values in research bioethics, health-care ethics consultation, and public policy bioethics. It makes no sense to be simultaneously a profession that tries to influence what those values should be in the public sphere. If they were to do so, it would result in a loss of legitimacy like lawyers would face if half of them took up dentistry while still calling themselves "lawyers." Government bioethics commissions should also end one of their common functions, "speaking to the public," because that is trying to simultaneously represent that public and change its views. It also violates the spirit of a liberal democratic society for the government to try to foster particular values in its citizens, instead of having the values of the citizens influence the government.

Moreover, since the bioethicists' principles would be from the public, having bioethicists advocate that the current public's values should be the future public's values is not only deeply conservative, it does not allow for the debate about ends that has so concerned social theorists. This practice would create the assumed ends that leads to Kass's concern about a slavish society.

This is not a call for the mass layoffs of bioethicists who want to promote their own values in the public sphere. When engaged in debates in research bioethics, health-care ethics consultation, or public policy bioethics, they would call themselves "bioethicists" and use either the existing principlist system for the first two, or my reformed principlist system for public policy bioethics. When engaged in debates in cultural bioethics, they could advocate for principles or values outside of those established to be already held by the public, as long as they used a different professional identity, like "philosopher."

This switching of identities is not as problematic as it sounds. Indeed, the bioethics profession already presumes that it can be done. The policy paper for the American Society for Bioethics and the Humanities concerning competencies in health-care ethics consultation calls for bioethicists who have another professional job in the hospital such as physician, nurse, or chaplain, when acting in their "role" as a bioethicist, to try to suppress their other role.[8] Similarly, former staff members of bioethics commissions have described changing their system of abstract knowledge from their usual academic philosophical one in order to fit with their new role (Dzur and Levin 2004:345–47).

Relocating the "Consensus Among Professionals" Method

So far, I have described cultural bioethical debate as if scholars emitted their thoughts into the ether. However, the founders of bioethical debate, like Daniel Callahan, have always called for direct debate among people of diverse intellectual perspectives who are engaging in what I have been calling *condensed translation* of their particular values.

I would transfer this method into the cultural bioethics task-space. I would hope that the institutions devoted toward bringing people of diverse values together to discuss issues could continue, albeit not under the aegis of the government. For example, the Hastings Center often has discussion meetings involving specific topics with people of varied professions and fairly varied points of view. The point is not to constrain conversation to what the public thinks, but to determine what the public should think, and to suggest these conclusions to the public, with the participants' views being honed through interaction. Similarly, the President's Council on Bioethics thought of itself as bringing together people of diverse perspectives so that they could enlighten each other, and its results were published in a series of books. My hope would be that something like this group could continue under the aegis of some private entity like a think tank, and that the participants would show each other where they are right and wrong, with the results influencing the thinking of the general public.

Bioethical Contributions to the Debate About Reproductive Cloning

Let us walk through a debate using the existing and proposed methods for bioethical debate. In the existing bioethics practice, the president might ask a standing government ethics commission to make a recommendation of ethical policy for reproductive cloning. The panel would think through and debate the issue and see how the four existing principles—autonomy, beneficence, non-maleficence, and justice—applied to this technology. This would mix with another method such as the "consensus among diverse commissioners" method. They would come to a recommendation and explicitly or implicitly say it was based on the shared values of the American people. The bioethics commission of the Clinton presidency did exactly this, and concluded that reproductive cloning should not be supported by the government because it potentially violated the principle of non-maleficence. Commissioners could not reach consensus on other concerns, so they were not considered further.

The implication, of course, is that if reproductive cloning were to become safe, then it would be acceptable to the panel. People might rightly wonder whether the four principles they used were actually the four principles of Americans, or whether they are the four principles favored by bioethicists and scientists. They might also wonder why the principles would be the same for reproductive cloning as for research on human subjects or the decision to end life support in a hospital. They might not recognize their values in any way the commission talked.

Other bioethicists would be engaged in cultural bioethics—talking to the *New York Times*, speaking on television, or teaching. Some would be promoting the four principles as what the public already believed, without evidence that this is the case, while implicitly claiming that, because the public believes this they should continue to believe this. Others would be promoting their own values or principles based on what they thought was right. People identified as bioethicists might be saying that reproductive cloning is ethically acceptable because it is an important value for humans to perfect ourselves. Others, citing the four principles, might say that the principle of autonomy leads us to the conclusion that, if people want to create cloned children, then they should be able to.

People might begin to wonder: Are these bioethicists representing the public's common values, or their own values?

In my proposed method, the president asks a standing government ethics commission to recommend an ethical policy for reproductive cloning. The panel commissions a team of social scientists who conduct various studies of the ends that the public would like to pursue with regard to the issue of reproductive cloning. The social scientists discover that five principles offer a good summary of the public's views: autonomy, beneficence, keeping people they way they are now, justice, and non-disturbance of "nature." The bioethicists on the panel publicize the results of the social-scientific analysis of the public, and turn to trying to come to an ethical recommendation; except that this is much harder than the similar process engaged in during the Clinton presidency, as some of the principles seem totally incommensurable. Conflicting principles cannot be ignored, as particular commissioners have been appointed to represent them. The commission cannot come to a solution given the divided nature of the public's values. Bioethicists across the country publish countless papers arguing that they have found a solution while those on the commission did not.

Is this gridlock worse than the previous situation? I would argue that it is better, as it more accurately reflects the values of the public. No consensual policy can be offered at this time, and I imagine that policy having to do with embryos might end up the same way. But this is a more democratic and publicly legitimate outcome than creating policy recommendations that purport to be based on everyone's values when (we would now know) they are not. If the commission were to evaluate research on human subjects, I suspect they would come up with more or less what is used now—not all issues would result in deadlock. (I think that policy on organ donation would be more consensual.) Since the public policy bioethics debate has publicly determined the values they are forwarding on behalf of the citizens, attempts by opponents of the outcome to discredit the commission, and bioethicists more generally, would fail.

The Final Defeat of the Theological Profession?

To finally wrap up my historical narrative, bioethics debates started with theology defending itself from science, but when theology struck back and weakened the scientific/medical jurisdiction over ethics, it was the bioethics profession that came in to obtain the subordinate jurisdictions. I have been concerned with strengthening the jurisdictional claims of bioethicists, but does this also mean that my system is the death knell to the theological profession's aspirations in these jurisdictions?

On the surface, the answer is "yes" for the health-care ethics consultation, research bioethics, and public policy bioethics jurisdictions. Given that, in these jurisdictions, principles, values, or ends would be preset, this task would be of little interest to theologians. Theological knowledge would not be useful for the task of weighing and balancing predetermined principles and trying to apply them to particular acts (like a proposed experiment). Indeed, as I showed in the history of bioethical debate in chapters 1 and 2, when the debate took on these qualities so that it would articulate with the new providers of jurisdiction, theologians left the debate due to lack of interest. As for why, I will simply restate Gustafson's quip quoted earlier, that this sort of analysis seems to a theologian like asking: "Should one cut the power source to a respirator for patient Y whose circumstances are a, b and c? [which] is not utterly dissimilar to asking whether $8.20 an hour or $8.55 an hour ought to be paid to carpenter's helpers in Kansas City" (Gustafson 1978:387). Theology is about "bigger" or "more abstract" issues than these, such as determining what the ends of a society should be. So, theologians would not and should not compete for jurisdiction over these tasks.

However, values of the religious component of the population will be better represented in these three jurisdictions in my system than they have been previously, because religious values are more likely to survive my translation than the transmutation currently used by bioethicists. Imagine, hypothetically, that all religious people believe that the current genetic composition of humans should not be changed, but that no non-religious person believes this. Given that, depending on how one counts, "religious" people are between 50 and 90 percent of the U.S. population, this value will be identified by social scientists and thus necessarily used by bioethicists. Using the current practice, the transmutation of this "religious" principle into the four existing principles cannot even be imagined (future people have not given their autonomous permission to be changed?). So, in theory my method would ensure that religious voices are represented according to their proportion in the general population.

By explicitly giving up on the first three jurisdictions, theologians can quite explicitly focus on their work in cultural bioethics. Nearly everyone accepts that theologians can say what they want in the public sphere to try to form public opinion—whether or not the people listen is of course another story. I would argue that it is imperative that theologians continue their efforts in public bioethics in that religion is a particularly rich source of values compared to other forms of discourse, and for a healthy public sphere we must have a debate about what our values should be.

I have obliquely mentioned throughout the book that bioethics has been competing for jurisdiction in cultural bioethics, and I would argue that it has been competing against theology, which is probably still in one of the strongest positions. If we were to ask the public the question: "which profession helps us understand the meaning of life and the purposes for which we humans should be working," the answer would probably be "the theology profession" or "the philosophy profession." These "big questions" are part of cultural bioethical debate, and theology should continue to debate the answers to these big questions. It is only with a public answer to the "big questions" can we get to the "smaller question" of whether a particular technology is consistent with or maximizes our values, and whether it should then be allowed.

Notes

1. The most influential opponent of this statement would be John Robertson, who would claim that many aspects of human reproduction are constitutionally protected in the same way that the right to abortion is (Robertson 1994; Robertson 2003; Robertson 2004). If he is correct, then these issues should not be matters of public policy bioethics anyway, because they are matters of individual conscience. (They would still be debated in cultural bioethics.)

2. This is a key statement in their article. However, I am guessing a bit that these two words in the bracket are what the authors intended to write, as there is a copy-editing error in the text. The text as printed is: "Discursive representation may, then do a morally superior because more comprehensive job of representing persons than do theories that treat individuals as unproblematic wholes."

3. For a good summary of these various mechanisms, see: http://www.cpn.org/tools/dictionary/deliberate.html.

4. Political scientists Albert Dzur and Daniel Levin agree on the usefulness of data on the public's views for public policy bioethics. They write that

> it is certainly possible to discover how people in different walks of life confront ethical problems and to delineate a range of possible approaches while clearly ruling out others with little standing in American moral discourse. Such information about Americans' moral reasoning is invaluable if commission reports are to inform general public debate. Concretely, one way of addressing public ways of moral decision making is for a commission to request extensive qualitative studies of actual moral deliberation (Dzur and Levin 2004:350).

5. On the details of the creation of the Belmont Report, which was part of the creation of the principles, see the competing accounts of Jonsen (2005) and Beauchamp (2005).

6. Kass, "New Beginnings in Life," 14.

7. Kass, "New Beginnings in Life," 16. This paragraph is taken from Evans (2002:64).

8. Per the American Society for Bioethics and Humanities:

> When an ethics consultant who is also a health care professional (e.g., physician, nurse, social worker, chaplain) is playing the

role of ethics consultant in a formal meeting, she should intro-
duce herself as an ethics consultant and explain that in that role
she is not acting as primary decision-maker, care provider, or
clinical consultant. Even when the clinical or professional expertise of the consultant is relevant to the case, the consultant
should refrain from providing clinical advice, but rather, defer
those decisions to the clinicians/professionals charged with
caring for the patient. Likewise, when an ethics case consultation is requested for a patient the consultant is caring for in her
"other" professional capacity (e.g., chaplain), then she should
enlist the involvement of another ethics consultant and clearly
explain to colleagues that she is there solely as the patient's
chaplain (American Society for Bioethics and Humanities
2011:19–20).

Chapter 6

Conclusion

Public policy bioethics is slowly evolving toward using interest-group legitimation, where social-movement activists, acting through political parties, provide ethical advice to government entities. Liberal bioethicists claim that the Republicans started this when Bush appointed a "partisan" group to his government bioethics committee. Republicans would probably retort that they were simply correcting the liberal bias of all previous bioethics appointees.

Liberals are setting up liberal bioethics institutions to counter what they see as the growing dominance of the conservatives (Charo 2007:104), and the Obama administration clearly is going to put its own preferred ethicists into the policy process. In the future, it seems that, if the Republicans win, then bioethicists who represent a particular evangelical, traditionalist Catholic, neo-conservative base of the Republican Party will get to recommend ethical policy. If the Democrats win, then the bioethicists who represent the scientific and medical establishment, along with religious liberals and secular people, will get the authority to recommend ethical policy. Bioethical recommendations are now increasingly dependent upon who wins the presidential election, not on any academic, professional deliberative process.

The Bioethicists' Response to the Crisis

The response of bioethicists to the crisis has largely been to ignore it. The liberal and conservative bioethicists seem to simply be arguing about who really represents the public's values, without acknowledging that the argument itself brings up the question of how any of them represent the public's values. There seems to be no recognition by either side that repeatedly pointing out that your challengers disagree with your ethical interpretations implies that your ethical interpretations cannot be based on a common morality. This further deepens the crisis for the profession.

This book advocates using new methods in the system of abstract knowledge of the bioethics profession. The bioethicists who also argue about the proper methods and the proper system of abstract knowledge of the profession—who in other fields would be called theorists—continue to write as if jurisdiction were granted by the American Philosophical Association. Many proposals for reforming bioethics presume that bioethics is primarily an academic field, and argue that attention to a new academic insight will improve the acceptance of the final product. For example, Howard Brody argues that a new "conceptual model . . . derived from one form of feminist ethics" should be applied to new areas of debate in bioethics (Brody 2009:105). Others argue for pragmatism, narrative, ethnographic, or other reforms. While I do not dispute that bioethical arguments could be improved in academic quality by taking advantage of insights from new academic sources, the source of the crisis in the bioethics profession is not that bioethics is not up to academic standards. Making bioethics academically "better" by making it more dependent on pragmatist philosophy will not increase its legitimacy in the eyes of the jurisdiction-givers, unless we have evidence that pragmatism will fill a need of these jurisdiction-givers.

Solving the Crisis by Focusing on the Needs of the Jurisdiction-Givers

What is occurring in the bioethics profession is not unique. Professions face jurisdictional crises all the time. If one were looking for a profession that has been in such crises repeatedly, one need look no further than theology. The entire literature on secularization is essentially the history of the endless jurisdictional crises of the theology profession as institution after institution has been removed from its control. Western governments were once under its jurisdiction—now gone. Higher education—gone. Family behavior—largely gone. On the other hand, some professions have caused crises for others. Medicine is probably the most successful profession, taking away the jurisdictions of others right and left in a process sociologists call "medicalization." Alcoholism and obesity, once considered moral failings, are now considered diseases, although the medical profession's jurisdiction over these new areas is not yet solid.

The bioethics profession is very new, and this is its first crisis. This is entirely predictable if we look at the history of professions. Professions start their jurisdiction with a system of abstract knowledge that fits the tasks quite well. Inevitably, the jurisdiction-provider changes, and the system of abstract knowledge designed for the task does not fit so well. For example, when public jurisdiction-givers came to accept modern psychology, the clergy began to lose jurisdiction over counseling people with marital problems. This change leaves the jurisdiction vulnerable to attack. Indeed, this is what has happened with the bioethics profession, as the government employees who use the ethical product and thus provide jurisdiction came to see bioethics as illegitimate because the religious right was pushing their bosses to be responsive to the religious right's values.

Nobody is challenging bioethics' primacy in the home jurisdictions of research bioethics and healthcare ethics consultation, but the challengers are attacking public policy bioethics by claiming that the bioethical system of abstract knowledge, when applied to public policy bioethics, is inaccurate. This is akin to dietary professionals' saying that the bariatric surgery of the medical profession does not actually work to alleviate obesity.

There are two responses to such a challenge. The first is retreat to the safer jurisdiction. The scientists who wanted to compete with theology for the task of determining the meaning and purpose of life did not make this challenge for long, and quickly retreated to their home jurisdiction of developing factual claims about the natural world. Retreat is a good strategy because, if you allow your profession to be discredited in an ancillary jurisdiction, it can weaken its reputation in other, more secure jurisdictions. This is what the scientists were worried about: that their jurisdictional expansion into the meaning and purpose of life would result in a public backlash in the scientists' more secure jurisdictions.

Another response to such a challenge is to change the system of abstract knowledge so that it better fits with both the secure and the threatened jurisdictions. If such a change would weaken the hold over the home jurisdiction, retreat is advised. This certainly would have fit science in the 1960s, as it is hard to imagine a system of abstract knowledge that would allow them strong jurisdiction both over the meaning and purpose of life *and* over explaining the functions of the physical world. Retreat was perhaps inevitable.

In other cases, new methods in the system of abstract knowledge can be created for both the safe and the threatened jurisdictions without damaging the hold over the home jurisdiction. That is what I am advocating in this book. The tasks in the research bioethics and health-care ethics consultation jurisdictions are set up so that the methods used in these jurisdictions are specific versions of a more general method used for public policy bioethics. That is, research bioethics and health-care ethics consultation are simply specific issues wherein the principles of the public can be determined empirically. This slight tweaking of the methods in the system of abstract knowledge will allow for secure jurisdiction over research bioethics, health-care ethics consultation, and public policy bioethics. Also key is that my proposal, while changing the methods, retains the system of abstract knowledge of using the values of others to derive ethics.

To defend the three jurisdictions, the bioethics profession must police its membership more stringently. At the most basic level, bioethicists are those who use the values of others to determine what is ethical, so people who call themselves "bioethicists" who are engaged in promoting their own values in cultural bioethics have to stop calling themselves bioethicists.

It is not possible to create one system of abstract knowledge that simultaneously uses the values of the public and tells the public what their values should be. Therefore, retreat from cultural bioethics is required. While such changes may seem painful, if you look at the history of the professions, such changes have always occurred. It is better to anticipate and plan for them instead of just letting your profession be delegitimized by others. This is simply part of "professionalization"—creating a more coherent profession.

Social-Movement Activists Will Not Immediately Go Away

I do not anticipate that bioethicists will be able to easily defeat social-movement activists for full jurisdiction in public policy bioethics. The right-to-life movement, the pro-choice movement, the scientific interest groups, the disease interest groups, the biotech industry associations, the pro- and anti-euthanasia groups, and more will all still be providing decision makers with ethical advice. My hope would be that with the profession of bioethics truly and transparently representing the common morality, it could show the other groups to be the interest groups that they are. I think that at least a faction, and hopefully a growing faction, could see the product of the bioethics profession as a way out of the polarized conflict of elites, and that elected officials would then have to justify why they are selecting the values of some of their constituents over the general values of the vast majority of them.

Utopias and Think-Pieces

I have made very specific and probably controversial proposals, and numerous oxen have been gored. I am under no illusion that my proposal will be recommended whole-cloth at the next meeting of the American Society for Bioethics and the Humanities. I am also under no illusion that social scientists are going to be asked by prominent bioethicists any time soon to determine what the values of society actually are for a given technology. Rather, the best outcome would be a debate about the points I raise. Change in the bioethics profession is going to have to come from within, with the ownership of the bioethics professionals. I hope to contribute to part of an internal reform effort that may not only save the jurisdictions of the bioethics profession, but may also retain a positive bioethical debate so that we as a society can face the biomedical challenges ahead.

WORKS CITED

Abbott, Andrew. 1988. *The System of Professions: An Essay on the Division of Expert Labor*. Chicago, IL: University of Chicago Press.

Advisory Committee on Human Radiation Experiments. 1996. *Final Report of the Advisory Committee on Human Radiation Experiments*. New York: Oxford University Press.

American Society for Bioethics and Humanities. 2011. *Report of the ASBH Core Competencies for Health Care Ethics Consultation (2nd edition)*. Glenview, IL: American Society for Bioethics and the Humanities.

Anspach, Renee R. 2010. "The 'Hostile Takeover' of Bioethics by Religious Conservatives and the Counter Offensive." Pp. 144–166 in *Social Movements and the Transformation of American Health Care*, edited by J. C. Banaszak-Hol, S. Levitsky, and M. N. Zald. New York: Oxford University Press.

Attwood, David. 1992. *Paul Ramsey's Political Ethics*. Lanham, MD: Rowman and Littlefield.

Baker, Robert. 2009. "In Defense of Bioethics." *Journal of Law, Medicine and Ethics* 37(1):83–92.

Banchoff, Thomas. 2011. *Embryo Politics: Ethics and Policy in Atlantic Democracies*. Ithaca, NY: Cornell University Press.

Beauchamp, Tom L. 1982. "What Philosophers Can Offer." *The Hastings Center Report* 12(3):13–14.

_____. 1995. "Principlism and Its Alleged Competitors." *Kennedy Institute of Ethics Journal* 5(3):181–198.

_____. 2005. "The Origins and Evolution of the Belmont Report." Pp. 12–25 in *Belmont Revisited: Ethical Principles for Research with Human Subjects*, edited by J. F. Childress, E. M. Meslin, and H. T. Shapiro. Washington, DC: Georgetown University Press.

Beauchamp, Tom L., and James F. Childress. 2001. *Principles of Biomedical Ethics*. 5. New York: Oxford University Press.

_____. 2009. *Principles of Biomedical Ethics (6th edition)*. New York: Oxford University Press.

Belkin, Gary S. 2004. "Moving Beyond Bioethics: History and the Search for Medical Humanism." *Perspectives in Biology and Medicine* 47(3):372–385.

Bellah, Robert N., Richard Madsen, William M. Sullivan, Ann Swidler, and Steven M. Tipton. 1985. *Habits of the Heart: Individualism and Commitment in American Life*. New York: Harper and Row.

Borry, Pascal, Paul Schotsmans, and Kris Dierickx. 2005. "The Birth of the Empirical Turn in Bioethics." *Bioethics* 19:49–71.

Bosk, Charles L. 1999. "Professional Ethicist Available: Logical, Secular, Friendly." *Daedalus*. 128 (4): 47–68.

Bosk, Charles L. 2008. *What Would You Do? Juggling Bioethics and Ethnography*. Chicago, IL: University of Chicago Press.

_____. 2010. "Bioethics, Raw and Cooked: Extraordinary Conflict and Everyday Practice." *Journal of Health and Social Behavior* 51(S):S133–S146.

Bosk, Charles L., and Raymond G. DeVries. 2004. "Bureaucracies of Mass Deception: IRBs and the Ethics of Ethnographic Research." *The Annals of the American Academy of Political and Social Science* 595(1):249–263.

Briggle, Adam. 2009. "The Kass Council and the Politicization of Ethics Advice." *Social Studies of Science* 39(2):309–326.

Brody, Baruch, Nancy Dubler, Jeff Blustein, Arthur Caplan, Jeffrey P. Kahn, Nancy Kass, Bernard Lo, Jonathan Moreno, Jeremy Sugarman, and Laurie Zoloth. 2002. "Bioethics Consultation in the Private Sector." *The Hastings Center Report* 32(3):14–20.

Brody, Howard. 2009. *The Future of Bioethics*. New York: Oxford University Press.

Brown, Mark B. 2009. "Three Ways to Politicize Bioethics." *American Journal of Bioethics*, 9(2):43–54.

Bulger, Ruth Ellen, Elizabeth Meyer Bobby, and Harvey V. Fineberg. 1995. *Society's Choices: Social and Ethical Decision Making in Biomedicine*. Washington, D.C.: National Academy Press.

Cahill, Lisa Sowle. 2005. *Theological Bioethics: Participation, Justice, Change*. Washington, DC: Georgetown University Press.

Callahan, Daniel. 1972. "New Beginnings in Life: A Philosopher's Response." Pp. 90–106 in *The New Genetics and the Future of Man*, edited by M. P. Hamilton. Grand Rapids, MI: Eerdmans Publishing Company.

_____. 1982. "At the Center." *Hastings Center Report* 12 (2): 4.

_____. 1990. "Religion and the Secularization of Bioethics." *The Hastings Center Report* 20 (4): 2–4.

_____. 1996. "Bioethics, Our Crowd, and Ideology." *Hastings Center Report* 26(6):3–4.

_____. 1999. "The Social Sciences and the Task of Bioethics." *Daedalus* 128(4):275–294.

_____. 2005. "Bioethics and the Culture Wars." *Cambridge Quarterly of Healthcare Ethics* 14:424–431.

_____. 2006. "Bioethics and Ideology." *Hastings Center Report* 36(1):3.

Campbell, Courtney S. 1993. "On James F. Childress: Answering That God in Every Person." Pp. 127–156 in *Theological Voices in Medical Ethics*, edited by A. Verhey and S. E. Lammers. Grand Rapids, MI: William B. Eerdmans.

_____. 1997. "Prophecy and Policy." *The Hastings Center Report* 27(5):15–17.

Caplan, Arthur L. 2005. "'Who Lost China?' A Foreshadowing of Today's Ideological Disputes in Bioethics." *Hastings Center Report* 35(3): 12–13.

_____. 2010. "Can Bioethics Transcend Ideology? (And Should It?)" Pp. 219–224 in *Progress in Bioethics: Science, Policy and Politics*, edited by J. Moreno and S. Berger. Cambridge, MA: MIT Press.

Capron, Alexander Morgan. 1983. "Looking Back at the President's Commission." *The Hastings Center Report* 13 (5) :7–10.

_____. 1989. "Bioethics on the Congressional Agenda." *Hastings Center Report* 19(March/April):22–23.

Carruthers, Bruce G., and Wendy Nelson Espeland. 1991. "Accounting for Rationality: Double-Entry Bookkeeping and the Rhetoric of Economic Rationality." *American Journal of Sociology* 97(1):31–69.

Centeno, Miguel Angel. 1997. *Democracy Within Reason: Technocratic Revolution in Mexico (2nd edition)*. University Park, PA: Pennsylvania State University Press.

Charo, R. Alta. 2004. "Passing on the Right: Conservative Bioethics Is Closer Than It Appears." *Journal of Law, Medicine and Ethics* 32:307–314.

_____. 2007. "The Endarkenment." Pp. 95–107 in *The Ethics of Bioethics: Mapping the Moral Landscape*, edited by L. A. Eckenwiler and F. G. Cohn. Baltimore, MD: The Johns Hopkins University Press.

Childress, James F. 1997. "The Challenges of Public Ethics: Reflections on NBAC's Report." *Hastings Center Report* 27(5):9–11.

_____. 2003. "Religion, Theology and Bioethics." Pp. 43–67 in *The Nature and Prospect of Bioethics*, edited by F. G. Miller, J. C. Fletcher, and J. M. Humber. Totowa, NJ: Humana Press.

Chisholm, Brock. 1963. "Future of the Mind." Pp. 315–321 in *Man and His Future*, edited by G. Wolstenholme. Boston: Little, Brown and Company.

Clouser, K. Danner. 1993. "Bioethics and Philosophy." *Hastings Center Report* 23(6):S10–11.

Clouser, K. Danner, and Bernard Gert. 1990. "A Critique of Principlism." *Journal of Medicine and Philosophy* 15:219–236.

Cohen, Cynthia B. 2005. "Promises and Perils of Public Deliberation: Contrasting Two National Bioethics Commissions on Embryonic Stem Cell Research." *Kennedy Institute of Ethics Journal* 15(3): 269–288.

Conrad, Peter. 2007. *The Medicalization of Society: On the Transformation of Human Conditions Into Treatable Disorders*. Baltimore, MD: Johns Hopkins University Press.

Cooter, Roger. 2004. "Historical Keywords: Bioethics." *The Lancet* 364:1749.

Cranford, Ronald E., and A. Edward Doudera. 1984. "The Emergence of Institutional Ethics Committees." *Law, Medicine and Health Care* 12(1):13–20.

Davidson, James D. 1994. "Religion Among America's Elite: Persistence and Change in the Protestant Establishment." *Sociology of Religion* 55(4):419–440.

Davidson, James D., Ralph E. Pyle, and David V. Reyes. 1995. "Persistence and Change in the Protestant Establishment." *Social Forces* 74(1):157–175.

Davis, Bernard D. 1970. "Prospects for Genetic Intervention in Man." *Science* 170:1279–1283.

Davis, James A., Tom W. Smith, and Peter V. Marsden. 2008. *General Social Survey, 1972-2008: Cumulative Codebook.* Chicago, IL: NORC.

Debruin, Debra A. 2007. "Ethics on the Inside?" Pp. 161–169 in *The Ethics of Bioethics: Mapping the Moral Landscape,* edited by L. A. Eckenwiler and F. G. Cohn. Baltimore, MD: The Johns Hopkins University Press.

Devettere, Raymond. 1995. "The Principled Approach: Principles, Rules and Actions." Pp. 27–48 in *Meta Medical Ethics: The Philosophical Foundations of Bioethics,* edited by M. A. Grodin. Dordrecht, The Netherlands: Kluwer Academic Publishers.

DeVries, Raymond. 2003. "How Can We Help? From 'Sociology in' to 'Sociology of' Bioethics." *Journal of Law, Medicine and Ethics* 32:1–14.

DeVries, Raymond, Leslie Rott, and Yasaswi Paruchuri. 2011. "Normative Environments of International Science." Pp. 105–120 in *International Research Collaborations: Much to Be Gained, Many Ways to Get in Trouble,* edited by M. S. Anderson and N. H. Steneck. New York: Routledge.

DeVries, Raymond, and Janardan Subedi. 1998. *Bioethics and Society: Constructing the Ethical Enterprise.* Upper Saddle River, NJ: Prentice Hall.

DeVries, Rob, and Bert Gordijn. 2009. "Empirical Ethics and Its Alleged Meta-Ethical Fallacies." *Bioethics* 23:193–201.

Dingwall, Robert. 2007. "'Turn Off the Oxygen....'" *Law and Society Review* 41(4):787–795.

Dryzek, John S., and Simon Niemeyer. 2008. "Discursive Representation." *American Political Science Review* 102(4):481–493.

DuBose, Edwin R., Ronald P. Hamel, and Laurence J. O'Connell. 1994. "Introduction." Pp. 1–17 in *A Matter of Principles? Ferment in U.S. Bioethics,* edited by E. R. DuBose, R. P. Hamel, and L. J. O'Connell. Valley Forge, PA: Trinity Press International.

Dzur, Albert W. 2002. "Democratizing the Hospital: Deliberative-Democratic Bioethics." *Journal of Health Politics, Policy and Law* 27(2):177–211.

_____. 2008. *Democratic Professionalism: Citizen Participation and the Reconstruction of Professional Ethics, Identity and Practice.* University Park, PA: Pennsylvania State University Press.

Dzur, Albert W., and Daniel Levin. 2004. "The 'Nation's Conscience': Assessing Bioethics Commissions as Public Forums." *Kennedy Institute of Ethics Journal* 14(4):333–360.

Ebbesen, Mette, and Birthe D. Pedersen. 2007. "Using Empirical Research to Formulate Normative Ethical Principles in Biomedicine." *Medicine, Health Care and Philosophy* 10:33–48.

Eckenwiler, Lisa A., and Felicia G. Cohn. 2007. "Introduction." Pp. xix–xx in *The Ethics of Bioethics: Mapping the Moral Landscape*, edited by L. A. Eckenwiler and F. G. Cohn. Baltimore, MD: The Johns Hopkins University Press.

Edwards, Robert G., and David J. Sharpe. 1971. "Social Values and Research in Human Embryology." *Nature* 231(14/May):87–91.

Edwards, Robert. 1989. *Life Before Birth: Reflections on the Embryo Debate*. New York: Basic Books.

Edwards, Robert, and Patrick Steptoe. 1980. *A Matter of Life: The Story of a Medical Breakthrough*. London: Hutchinson.

Elliott, Carl. 2004. "Beyond Politics: Why Have Bioethicists Focused on the President's Council's Dismissals and Ignored Its Remarkable Work?" *Slate*, 25/March. http://www.slate.com/id/2096815/

———. 2005. "The Soul of the New Machine: Bioethicists in the Bureaucracy." *Cambridge Quarterly of Healthcare Ethics* 14:379–384.

———. 2007. "The Tyranny of Expertise." Pp. 43–46 in *The Ethics of Bioethics: Mapping the Moral Landscape*, edited by L. A. Eckenwiler and F. G. Cohn. Baltimore, MD: The Johns Hopkins University Press.

Engelhardt, H. Tristram. 1986. *The Foundations of Bioethics*. New York: Oxford University Press.

———. 2000. *The Foundations of Christian Bioethics*. Exton, PA: Swets and Zeitlinger.

———. 2007. "Bioethics as Politics: A Critical Reassessment." Pp. 118–133 in *The Ethics of Bioethics: Mapping the Moral Landscape*, edited by L. A. Eckenwiler and F. G. Cohn. Baltimore, MD: The Johns Hopkins University Press.

Espeland, Wendy Nelson. 1998. *The Struggle for Water: Politics, Rationality, and Identity in the American Southwest*. Chicago, IL: University of Chicago Press.

Espeland, Wendy Nelson, and Mitchell L. Stevens. 1998. "Commensuration as a Social Process." *Annual Review of Sociology* 24: 313–331.

Evans, John H. 2002. *Playing God? Human Genetic Engineering and the Rationalization of Public Bioethical Debate*. Chicago, IL: University of Chicago Press.

_____. 2010. *Contested Reproduction: Genetic Technologies, Religion, and Public Debate*. Chicago, IL: University of Chicago Press.

Evans, John H., and Michael S. Evans. 2008. "Religion and Science: Beyond the Epistemological Conflict Narrative." *Annual Review of Sociology* 2008:87–105.

Evans, Michael S., and John H. Evans. 2010. "Arguing Against Darwinism: Religion, Science and Public Morality." Pp. 286–308 in *The New Blackwell Companion to the Sociology of Religion*, edited by B. Turner. New York: Blackwell.

Ezrahi, Yaron. 1990. *The Descent of Icarus: Science and the Transformation of Contemporary Democracy*. Cambridge, MA: Harvard University Press.

Faden, Ruth R., and Tom L. Beauchamp. 1986. *A History and Theory of Informed Consent*. New York: Oxford University Press.

Feeley, Malcolm M. 2007. "Legality, Social Research, and the Challenge of Institutional Review Boards." *Law and Society Review* 41(4):757–776.

Fischer, Frank. 1990. *Technocracy and the Politics of Expertise*. Newbury Park, CA: Sage Publications.

Fletcher, John C., Norman Quist, and Albert R. Jonsen. 1989. "Ethics Consultation in Health Care: Rationale and History." Pp. 1–15 in *Ethics Consultation in Health Care*, edited by J. C. Fletcher, N. Quist, and A. R. Jonsen. Ann Arbor, MI: Health Administration Press.

Fletcher, Joseph. 1954. *Morals and Medicine*. Princeton, NJ: Princeton University Press.

_____. 1966. *Situation Ethics: The New Morality*. Philadelphia, PA: Westminster Press.

_____. 1971. "Ethical Aspects of Genetic Controls." *New England Journal of Medicine* 285(14):776–783.

_____. 1993. "Memoir of an Ex-Radical." Pp. 55–92 in *Joseph Fletcher: Memoir of an Ex-Radical*, edited by K. Vaux. Louisville, KY: Westminster/John Knox.

Fox, Ellen, Kenneth A. Berkowitz, Barbara L. Chanko, and Tia Powell. 2006. *Ethics Consultation: Responding to Ethics Questions in Health Care*. Washington, D.C: Veterans Health Administration.

Fox, Ellen, Sarah Myers, and Robert A. Pearlman. 2007. "Ethics Consultation in United States Hospitals: A National Survey." *American Journal of Bioethics* 7(2):13–25.

Fox, Renée C., and Judith P. Swazey. 1984. "Medical Morality is not Bioethics—Medical Ethics in China and the United States." *Perspectives in Biology and Medicine* 27(3):336–360.

_____. 2008. *Observing Bioethics*. New York: Oxford University Press.

Gamerman, Ellen. 2001. "Bioethics Council Chief Said to Share Bush's View on Stem Cell Research." *The Baltimore Sun*, 11/August.

Green, Ronald M. 2001. *The Human Embyro Research Debates: Bioethics in the Vortex of Controversy*. New York: Oxford University Press.

Gustafson, James M. 1978. "Theology Confronts Technology and the Life Sciences." *Commonweal* 105:386–392.

Gutmann, Amy, and Dennis Thompson. 1996. *Democracy and Disagreement*. Cambridge, MA: Harvard University Press.

Hanna, Kathi E., Robert M. Cook-Deegan, and Robyn Y. Nishimi. 1993. "Finding a Forum for Bioethics in U.S. Public Policy." *Politics and the Life Sciences* 12(2):205–219.

Hanson, Mark J. 1999. "Lessons from a Religious Objection to Genetic Patenting." Pp. 221–234 in *Perspectives on Genetic Patenting: Religion, Science, and Industry in Dialogue*, edited by A. R. Chapman. Washington, D.C.: American Association for the Advancement of Science.

Harris, John. 2003. "In Praise of Unprincipled Ethics." *Journal of Medical Ethics* 29:303–306.

Hauerwas, Stanley M. 1997. *Wilderness Wanderings: Probing Twentieth-Century Theology and Philosophy*. Boulder, CO: Westview Press.

Hauerwas, Stanley. 1996. "How Christian Ethics Became Medical Ethics: The Case of Paul Ramsey." Pp. 61–80 in *Religion and Medical Ethics: Looking Back, Looking Forward*, edited by A. Verhey. Grand Rapids, MI: William B. Eerdmans.

Hedgecoe, Adam M. 2004. "Critical Bioethics: Beyond the Social Science Critique of Applied Ethics." *Bioethics* 18:120–143.

Hester, D. Micah. 2003. "Is Pragmatism Well-Suited to Bioethics?" *Journal of Medicine and Philosophy* 28(5–6):545–561.

Hoffmaster, Barry. 1991. "The Theory and Practice of Applied Ethics." *Dialogue* 30:213–234.

Hurlbut, James Benjamin. 2010. "Experiments in Democracy: The Science, Politics and Ethics of Human Embryo Research in the United States, 1978–2007." Ph.D. diss., History of Science, Harvard University.

Jasanoff, Sheila. 2005. *Designs on Nature: Science and Democracy in Europe and the United States*. Princeton, NJ: Princeton University Press.

Jensen, Eric. 2008. "Through Thick and Thin: Rationalizing the Public Bioethical Debate Over Therapeutic Cloning." *Clinical Ethics* 3: 194–198.

Johnson, Summer. 2006. "Multiple Roles and Successes in Public Bioethics: A Response to the Public Forum Critique of Bioethics Commissions." *Kennedy Institute of Ethics Journal* 16(2):173–188.

Jonsen, Albert R. 1994. "Foreword." Pp. ix–xvii in *A Matter of Principles? Ferment in U.S. Bioethics*, edited by E. R. DuBose, R. P. Hamel, and L. J. O'Connell. Valley Forge, PA: Trinity Press International.

———. 1998. *The Birth of Bioethics*. New York: Oxford University Press.

———. 2005. "On the Origins and Future of the Belmont Report." Pp. 3–11 in *Belmont Revisited: Ethical Principles for Research with Human Subjects*, edited by J. F. Childress, E. M. Meslin, and H. T. Shapiro. Washington, DC: Georgetown University Press.

———. 2006. "A History of Religion and Bioethics." Pp. 23–36 in *Handbook of Bioethics and Religion*, edited by D. E. Guinn. New York: Oxford University Press.

Jonsen, Albert R., Mark Siegler, and William J. Winslade. 2006. *Clinical Ethics: A Practical Approach to Ethical Decisions in Clinical Medicine (6th edition)*. New York: McGraw Hill.

Jonsen, Albert R., and Stephen Toulmin. 1988. *The Abuse of Casuistry: A History of Moral Reasoning*. Berkeley, CA: University of California Press.

Kass, Leon R. 1972. "New Beginnings in Life." Pp. 15–63 in *The New Genetics and the Future of Man*, edited by M. Hamilton. Grand Rapids, MI: Eerdmans.

———. 2005. "Reflections on Public Bioethics: A View from the Trenches." *Kennedy Institute of Ethics Journal* 15(3):221–250.

Katz, Jack. 2007. "Toward a Natural History of Ethical Censorship." *Law and Society Review* 41(4):797–810.

Kaye, Howard L. 1997. *The Social Meaning of Modern Biology: From Social Darwinism to Sociobiology*. New Brunswick, NJ: Transaction Publishers.

Kuczewski, Mark G. 2007. "Democratic Ideals and Bioethics Commissions: The Problem of Expertise in an Egalitarian Society." Pp. 83–94 in *The Ethics of Bioethics: Mapping the Moral Landscape*, edited by L. A. Eckenwiler and F. G. Cohn. Baltimore, MD: The Johns Hopkins University Press.

Lammers, Stephen E. 1996. "The Marginalization of Religious Voices in Bioethics." Pp. 19–43 in *Religion and Medical Ethics: Looking Back, Looking Forward*, edited by A. Verhey. Grand Rapids, MI: William B Eerdmans.

Laney, James T. 1970. "The New Morality and the Religious Communities." *The Annals of the American Academy of Political and Social Science* 387:14–21.

Lebacqz, Karen. 2005. "We Sure Are Older But Are We Wiser?" Pp. 99–110 in *Belmont Revisited: Ethical Principles for Research with Human Subjects*, edited by J. F. Childress, E. M. Meslin, and H. T. Shapiro. Washington, DC: Georgetown University Press.

Leget, Carlo, Pascal Borry, and Raymond DeVries. 2009. "'Nobody Tosses a Dwarf!' The Relation Between the Empirical and the Normative Reexamined." *Bioethics* 23:226–235.

Lillehammer, Hallvard. 2004. "Who Needs Bioethicists?" *Studies in the History and Philosophy of Biological and Biomedical Sciences* 35:131–144.

Long, D. Stephen. 1993. *Tragedy, Tradition, Transformism: The Ethics of Paul Ramsey*. Boulder, CO: Westview Press.

Lukes, Steven. 1974. *Power*. London: Macmillan.

Luria, S. E. 1965. "Directed Genetic Change: Perspectives from Molecular Genetics." Pp. 1–19 in *The Control of Human Heredity and Evolution*, edited by T. Sonneborn. New York: The Macmillan Company.

Lysaught, M. Therese. 2004. "Respect: Or, How Respect for Persons Became Respect for Autonomy." *Journal of Medicine and Philosophy* 29(6):665–680.

_____. 2006. "And Power Corrupts...: Religion and the Disciplinary Matrix of Bioethics." Pp. 93–128 in *Handbook of Bioethics and Religion*, edited by D. E. Guinn. New York: Oxford University Press.

Macklin, Ruth. 2006. "The New Conservatives in Bioethics: Who Are They and What Do They Seek?" *Hastings Center Report* 36(1): 34–43.

_____. 2010. "The Death of Bioethics (As We Once Knew It)." *Bioethics* 24(5):211–217.

MacNamara, Vincent. 1985. *Faith and Ethics: Recent Roman Catholicism*. Washington, DC: Georgetown University Press.

Marty, Martin. 1992. "Religion, Theology, Church, and Bioethics." *Journal of Medicine and Philosophy* 17:273–289.

May, William F. 2010. "Finding Common Ground in Bioethics?" Pp. 257–271 in *Progress in Bioethics: Science, Policy and Politics*, edited by J. Moreno and S. Berger. Cambridge, MA: MIT Press.

McGee, Glenn. 1999. *Pragmatic Bioethics*. Nashville, TN: Vanderbilt University Press.

Messikomer, Carla M., Renée C. Fox, and Judith P. Swazey. 2001. "The Presence and Influence of Religion in American Bioethics." *Perspectives in Biology and Medicine* 44(4):485–508.

Miller, Franklin G., Arthur L. Caplan, and John C. Fletcher. 1998. "Dealing with Dolly: Inside the National Bioethics Advisory Commission." *Health Affairs* 17(3):264–267.

Moen, Matthew C. 1992. *The Transformation of the Christian Right*. Tuscaloosa, AL: University of Alabama Press.

Moreno, Jonathan D. 1995. *Deciding Together: Bioethics and Moral Consensus*. New York: Oxford University Press.

_____. 2005. "The End of the Great Bioethics Compromise." *Hastings Center Report* 35(1):20–21.

Moreno, Jonathan D., and Sam Berger. 2010. *Progress in Bioethics: Science, Policy and Politics*. Cambridge, MA: MIT Press.

National Commission for the Protection of Human Subjects of Biomedical and Behavioral Research. 1978a. *The Belmont Report: Ethical Principles and Guidelines for the Protection of Human Subjects of Research*. Washington, DC: Government Printing Office.

_____. 1978b. *Special Study: Implications of Advances in Biomedical and Behavioral Research*. Washington, D.C: Government Printing Office.

Nature editorial. 2006. "Bioethics at the Bench: Bioethicists Should Be Close—But Not Too Close—to the Lab Action." *Nature* 440(7088):1089–1090.

Nelson, James Lindemann. 2005. "The Baroness's Committee and the President's Council: Ambition and Alienation in Public Bioethics." *Kennedy Institute of Ethics Journal* 15(3):251–267.

Noll, Mark A. 1992. *A History of Christianity in the United States and Canada*. Grand Rapids, MI: Eerdmans.

Pateman, Carole. 1970. *Participation and Democratic Theory*. Cambridge, UK: Cambridge University Press.

Pellegrino, Edmund D. 2006. "Bioethics and Politics: 'Doing Ethics' in the Public Square." *Journal of Medicine and Philosophy* 31:569–584.

Perrin, Andrew J., and Katherine McFarland. 2008. "The Sociology of Political Representation and Deliberation." *Sociological Compass* 2(4):1228–1244.

Perrow, Charles. 1986. *Complex Organizations: A Critical Essay, (3rd edition)*. New York: Random House.

Persad, Govind C., Linden Elder, Laura Sedig, Leonardo Flores, and Ezekiel J. Emanuel. 2008. "The Current State of Medical School Education in Bioethics, Health Law, and Health Economics." *Journal of Law, Medicine and Ethics* 36(1):89–94.

Porter, Theodore M. 1995. *Trust in Numbers: The Pursuit of Objectivity in Science and Public Life*. Princeton, NJ: Princeton University Press.

Post, Linda Farber, Jeffrey Blustein, and Nancy Neveloff Dubler. 2007. *Handbook of Health Care Ethics Committees*. Baltimore, MD: The Johns Hopkins University Press.

President's Commission for the Study of Ethical Problems in Medicine and Biomedical and Behavioral Research. 1982. *Making Health Care Decisions, The Ethical and Legal Implications of Informed Consent in the Patient–Practitioner Relationship. Volume Two: Appendices, Empirical Studies of Informed Consent*. Washington, D.C: Government Printing Office.

———. 1983a. *Deciding to Forego Life Sustaining Treatment: A Report on the Ethical, Medical and Legal Issues in Treatment Decisions*. Washington, D.C: Government Printing Office.

———. 1983b. *Splicing Life: A Report on the Social and Ethical Issues of Genetic Engineering with Human Beings*. Washington, D.C.: Government Printing Office.

———. 1983c. *Summing Up*. Washington, D.C.: Government Printing Office.

President's Council on Bioethics. 2003. *Beyond Therapy: Biotechnology and the Pursuit of Happiness*. Washington, DC: President's Council on Bioethics.

Ramsey, Paul. 1968. "The Morality of Abortion." Pp. 60–93 in *Life or Death: Ethics and Options*, edited by D. H. Labby. Seattle, WA: University of Washington Press.

———. 1970a. *Fabricated Man: The Ethics of Genetic Control*. New Haven, CT: Yale University Press.

———. 1970b. *The Patient as Person*. New Haven, CT: Yale University Press.

Rawls, John. 1993. *Political Liberalism*. New York: Columbia University Press.

Reich, Warren Thomas. 1995. "The Word 'Bioethics': The Struggle Over Its Earliest Meanings." *Kennedy Institute of Ethics Journal* 5(1):19–34.

Robertson, John A. 1994. *Children of Choice: Freedom and the New Reproductive Technologies*. Princeton, NJ: Princeton University Press.

———. 2003. "Procreative Liberty in the Era of Genomics." *American Journal of Law and Medicine* 29:439–487.

———. 2004. "Procreative Liberty and Harm to Offspring in Assisted Reproduction." *American Journal of Law and Medicine* 30:7–40.

Rosenberg, Charles E. 1999. "Meanings, Policies, and Medicine: On the Bioethical Enterprise and History." *Daedalus* 128(4):27–46.

Rothman, David J. 1991. *Strangers by the Bedside: A History of How Law and Bioethics Transformed Medical Decision Making*. New York: Basic Books.

Salter, Brian, and Mavis Jones. 2005. "Biobanks and Bioethics: The Politics of Legitimation." *Journal of European Public Policy* 12: 710–732.

Salter, Brian, and Charlotte Salter. 2007. "Bioethics and the Global Moral Economy: The Cultural Politics of Human Embryonic Stem Cell Science." *Science, Technology and Human Values* 32(5):554–581.

Scofield, Giles R. 2008. "What is Medical Ethics Consultation?" *Journal of Law, Medicine and Ethics* 36(1):95–118.

Shils, Edward. 1968. "The Sanctity of Life." Pp. 2–39 in *Life or Death: Ethics and Options*, edited by D. H. Labby. Seattle, WA: University of Washington Press.

Singer, Peter. 1982. "How Do We Decide?" *Hastings Center Report* 12(3):9–11.

Slowther, Anne. 2007. "Ethics Consultation and Ethics Committees." Pp. 527–534 in *Principles of Health Care Ethics (2nd edition)*, edited by R. E. Ashcroft, A. Dawson, H. Draper, and J. R. McMillan. West Sussex, UK: John Wiley and Sons.

Smith, Christian. 1998. *American Evangelicalism: Embattled and Thriving*. Chicago, IL: University of Chicago Press.

———. 2003. *The Secular Revolution*. Berkeley, CA: University of California Press.

Smith, David H. 1993. "On Paul Ramsey: A Covenant-Centered Ethic for Medicine." Pp. 7–29 in *Theological Voices in Medical Ethics*, edited by A. Verhey and S. E. Lammers. Grand Rapids, MI: William B. Eerdmans.

Stark, Laura. (2012). *Behind Closed Doors*. Chicago, IL: University of Chicago Press.

Steensland, Brian, Jerry Z. Park, Mark D. Regnerus, Lynn D. Robinson, W. Bradford Wilcox, and Robert D. Woodberry. 2000. "The Measure of American Religion: Toward Improving the State of the Art." *Social Forces* 79(1):291–318.

Taylor, Charles. 1995. "Liberal Politics and the Public Sphere." Pp. 183–217 in *The New Communitarian Thinking*, edited by A. Etzioni. Charlottesville, VA: University Press of Virginia.

Teel, Karen. 1975. "The Physician's Dilemma, a Doctor's View: What the Law Should Be." *Baylor Law Review* 27:6–9.

Thielicke, Helmut. 1970. "The Doctor as Judge of Who Shall Live and Who Shall Die." Pp. 146–186 in *Who Shall Live? Medicine, Technology, Ethics*, edited by K. Vaux. Philadelphia, PA: Fortress Press.

Tong, Rosemarie. 1997. *Feminist Approaches to Bioethics: Theoretical Reflections and Practical Applications*. Boulder, CO: Westview Press.

Trotter, Griffin. 2007. "Left Bias in Academic Bioethics." Pp. 95–107 in *The Ethics of Bioethics: Mapping the Moral Landscape*, edited by L. A. Eckenwiler and F. G. Cohn. Baltimore, MD: The Johns Hopkins University Press.

Tubbs, James B. 1996. *Christian Theology and Medical Ethics*. Dordrecht, The Netherlands: Kluwer Academic Publishers.

Turner, Leigh. 2003. "Zones of Consensus and Zones of Conflict: Questioning the 'Common Morality' Presumption in Bioethics." *Kennedy Institute of Ethics Journal* 13(3):193–218.

———. 2009. "Bioethics and Social Studies of Medicine: Overlapping Concerns." *Cambridge Quarterly of Healthcare Ethics* 18:36–42.

U.S. Congress, Office of Technology Assessment. 1993. *Biomedical Ethics in U.S. Public Policy—Background Paper*. Washington, DC: Government Printing Office.

Veatch, Robert M. 1977. "Hospital Ethics Committees: Is There a Role?" *Hastings Center Report* 7(3):22–25.

———. 2007. "How Many Principles for Bioethics?" Pp. 43–50 in *Principles of Healthcare Ethics*, edited by R. E. Ashcroft, A. Dawson, H. Draper, and J. R. McMillan. West Sussex, UK: John Wiley and Sons.

Verhey, Allen. 1995. "'Playing God' and Invoking a Perspective." *Journal of Medicine and Philosophy* 20:347–364.

Verhey, Allen, and Stephen E. Lammers. 1993. *Theological Voices in Bioethics*. Grand Rapids, MI: Eerdmans Publishing Company.

Walters, LeRoy. 1985. "Religion and the Renaissance of Medical Ethics in the United States." Pp. 3–16 in *Theology and Bioethics*, edited by E. Shelp. Boston, MA: D. Reidel Publishing Company.

Weber, Max. 1968. *Economy and Society (2 volumes)*. Berkeley, CA: University of California Press.

Wilcox, Clyde. 2009. "Of Movements and Metaphors: The Co-Evolution of the Christian Right and the GOP." Pp. 331–356 in *Evangelicals and Democracy in America. Volume II: Religion and Politics*, edited by S. Brint and J. Schroedel. New York: Russell Sage Foundation Press.

Wilde, Melissa J. 2007. *Vatican II: A Sociological Analysis of Religious Change*. Princeton, NJ: Princeton University Press.

Wilson, James Q. 1989. *Bureaucracy: What Government Agencies Do and Why They Do It*. New York: Basic Books.

Wolstenholme, Gordon. 1963. *Man and His Future*. Edited by G. Wolstenholme. London: J. & A. Churchill Ltd.

Wright, Susan. 1994. *Molecular Politics: Developing American and British Regulatory Policy for Genetic Engineering, 1972–1982*. Chicago: University of Chicago Press.

Wuthnow, Robert. 1988. *The Restructuring of American Religion*. Princeton, NJ: Princeton University Press.

Wuthnow, Robert, and John H. Evans. 2002. *The Quiet Hand of God: Faith-Based Activism and the Public Role of Mainline Protestantism*. Berkeley, CA: University of California Press.

Yearley, Steven. 2009. "The Ethical Landscape: Identifying the Right Way to Think About the Ethical and Societal Aspects of Synthetic Biology Research and Products." *Journal of the Royal Society Interface* 6(Suppl. 4): S559–S564.

Yoder, Scot D. 1998. "Experts in Ethics? The Nature of Ethical Expertise." *Hastings Center Report* 28(6):11–19.

INDEX

AARP (American Association of
  Retired Persons), *xii*
Abbott, Andrew, *xvii*, *xviii–xix*, 103
abstract knowledge. *see also*
  common morality
  principlism
  of bioethics profession, *xxii*,
    xxvi–xxvii, *xlviii*
  criticism of, *xlix* (n10)
  de-legitimized system of,
    xxxix–xl
  jurisdiction-givers and, *xlvi*
  President's Council on
    Bioethics and, 86–89
  professional jurisdiction and,
    xviii, *xxxviii*, *xliii*
  public-policy bioethics
    jurisdiction and, *xliv*
  subordination in, 103–104
academic reflection, 126
academic texts, *xxxii*
accommodation, 68–69n5
Advisory Committee on Human
  Radiation Experiments,
  135–136

advisory committees, 38–42.
  see also committees/
  commissions
advisory jurisdiction, 128n1
agape, 16–18, 30
agenda setting, *xiv*
American Association of Retired
  Persons (AARP), *xii*
American Society for Bioethics
  and the Humanities, *xvi*,
  102, 156, 162–163n8
analytic philosophy, 134–135
autonomous ethic
  theology, 25
autonomy, 71n15, 115

Bacon, Francis, 88, 122
Barth, Karl, 17, 20
Beauchamp, Tom
  on academic reflection,
    126–127
  on common-morality
    principlism, *l* (n 13), 45–47,
    51–52, 57
  form of argumentation, 64

Printed in Germany
by Amazon Distribution
GmbH, Leipzig